DID YOU KNOW?

- Nickel allergy is skyrocketing among teenagers, due to the growing popularity of navel piercing.

- Improved hygiene and childhood vaccinations may be causing allergies.

- Deadly food allergies are on the rise— between 5 and 10 percent of the population is allergic to common foods such as peanuts, shellfish, soy, and milk products.

- Indoor allergies—once rare—are now commonplace; allergies to dust mites and mold are a leading cause of asthma and chronic sinus infection.

- Chemicals found in latex gloves cause rashes and respiratory symptoms in up to 20 percent of all health professionals.

- New drugs trigger allergies—3 percent of all hospitalized patients will experience a severe allergic reaction to a new medication.

COMPREHENSIVE, AUTHORITATIVE, AND COMPLETELY CUTTING EDGE, THIS IS THE BOOK THAT CAN HELP YOU TAKE CONTROL OF YOUR ALLERGIES LIKE NEVER BEFORE…

EARL MINDELL'S ALLERGY BIBLE

Also by Dr. Earl Mindell

Dr. Mindell's Vitamin Bible for the 21st. Century

New Herb Bible

Parent's Nutrition Bible

Food as Medicine

Soy Miracle

Anti-Aging Bible

Secret Remedies

Supplement Bible

Prescription Alternatives

Peak Performance Bible

Diet Bible

Unsafe at any Meal: How to Avoid Hidden Toxins in Your Food

Dr. Earl Mindell's Natural Remedies for 101 Ailments

EARL MINDELL'S
ALLERGY
BIBLE

Includes Hundreds of Conventional and Alternative Strategies and Treatments for Every Kind of Allergy

EARL MINDELL, R.Ph., Ph.D.

WARNER BOOKS

An AOL Time Warner Company

WARNER BOOKS EDITION

Copyright © 2003 by Earl Mindell R.Ph., Ph.D., and Carol Colman
All rights reserved. No part of this book may be reproduced in any form or by any electronic or mechanical means, including information storage and retrieval systems, without permission in writing from the publisher, except by a reviewer who may quote brief passages in a review.

Cover design by Elaine Groh
Book design by Charles S. Sutherland

Warner Books, Inc.
1271 Avenue of the Americas
New York, NY 10020

Visit our Web site at www.twbookmark.com

 An AOL Time Warner Company

Printed in the United States of America

First Printing: April 2003

10 9 8 7 6 5 4 3 2 1

To my wife and soulmate, Gail, to our children, Alanna and Evan, to all my friends and family for their support, and to the millions nationwide who now have a vehicle for winning the battle against allergies and asthma, without using dangerous, harmful, and toxic substances.

Acknowledgments

I wish to express my deep and lasting appreciation to my friends and associates, who have assisted me in the preparation of this book, especially Howard Segal, Ph.D., Bernard Bubman, R.Ph., Alan Khasin, Ph.D., Stewart Fisher, M.D., Rory Jaffe, M.D., Donald Cruden, O.D., Raymond Faltinsky, J.D., and Kevin Fournier. I would also like to thank Carol Colman Gerber, agent Richard Curtis, and my editor John Aherne and his able assistant, Megan Rickman.

Contents

EARL
MINDELL'S
ALLERGY
BIBLE

CHAPTER 1

The Allergy Epidemic

IF YOU'RE READING THIS BOOK, CHANCES ARE THAT YOU or your loved ones suffer from allergies, asthma, or both. And chances are, you think that it's impossible to get through a day without taking over-the-counter or prescription drugs, particularly during allergy season. Some of you may worry that you are becoming overly dependent on strong medicines. You may even have tried to incorporate alternative therapies, such as vitamins, herbs, and other supplements, into your treatment regimen, but when you went to the pharmacy or natural food store to purchase them, you were overwhelmed by the volume of products on the shelves, and you didn't know how to select the right ones. If you are already using alternative therapies, you may not be sure that you are using them correctly, or that you are taking the best supplements for your problem. I am writing this book for you.

I am a pharmacist, master herbalist, and longtime student of alternative medicine. I am not against drugs, but believe in using them only when absolutely necessary. I believe that many cases of allergy and asthma can be managed successfully by making changes in lifestyle and diet, and by the judicious use of natural supplements. It is my goal to help you live as full, healthy, and drug-free a life as possible. Many of you with mild allergic symptoms will find that by following the advice in this book, you will be able to significantly reduce your need for drugs, or may no longer require them. Those of you with more serious forms of allergy and asthma may still need conventional medication, but you should see an improvement in your symptoms. At the very least, you will be taking charge of your health, and doing positive things that will not only relieve your asthma and allergy, but reduce your risk of developing many chronic diseases.

I have a personal stake in this book. Both my wife and son suffer from severe allergies, which are now being successfully treated with supplements and other alternative therapies. I know that these remedies can work if you know how to use them safely and effectively.

YOU'RE NOT ALONE

First, I'd like to tell you a bit about what allergy is, and why it has become one of the fastest-growing epidemics in history. If you lived one hundred years ago, chances are you would not be allergic, and, in fact, there would be no need for this book! At the dawn of the twentieth century, allergy was a mysterious and rare condition that affected only a tiny minority of people. Just a few generations later, allergy has become as common as the common cold. Despite the growing attempts of health-care professionals to control the allergy epidemic, it's growing worse.

About 30 percent of all adults and 40 percent of all children in the United States have hay fever, an allergy to plant pollen that torments sufferers from March through November. The incidence of asthma, a potentially serious lung condition most often triggered by allergy, has more than doubled since the 1980s, afflicting more than 15 million Americans.

About 5 percent of the population are allergic to common foods, such as peanuts, shellfish, milk, and even soy products. For some food allergy sufferers, exposure to even a microscopic amount of an offending substance can cause anaphylactic shock and even death.

Once rare, indoor allergies are on the rise, including allergies to dust mites, molds, and pets. No wonder! Today, people spend 90 percent of their time indoors. Allergies are rampant in the workplace. The proliferation of new chemicals and poorly ventilated "sick buildings" have triggered new allergies. A case in point: Nearly 12 percent of all medical workers who wear latex gloves (to prevent the spread of HIV and other infections) have developed serious allergies to latex!

New drugs are spawning new allergies. About 3 percent of all hospitalized patients will experience a severe allergic reaction to a new medication.

More than 50 million Americans are allergic to *something*. What exactly is allergy? And why is it on the rise?

First, there are a great many misconceptions about allergy that I would like to clear up. The primary one is that most people confuse their *symptoms* with their *allergies*. For example, if you have a runny, itchy nose, you may think your allergy is related to your respiratory system. Or, if you have hives, you may think that you have a skin condition, or if you have food allergies, you may think that your symptoms are due to a weak gastrointestinal system. In reality, regardless of where or how allergies may strike, all allergies stem from one system—your immune system. If you have an allergy, you have an immune problem.

ALLERGY IS AN IMMUNE SYSTEM PROBLEM

An allergy is an overreaction of the body's immune system to a normally harmless substance, such as plant pollen, wheat, animal dander, or a chemical. The offending substance can be inhaled through the mouth or nose, or can be swallowed, or can make contact with the skin. Unlike infection, allergy is not contagious and is not spread from person to person.

Where is your immune system, and why is it allergy prone? Your immune system is unique in that it isn't quickly identified with a particular organ as, for example, your heart is linked to your cardiovascular system or your brain to your nervous system. That's because your immune system is not confined to any one site in the body—it is everywhere. Your immune system is an assortment of billions of specialized cells that protect your body in many different ways. Immune cells are in the skin, the lungs, the eyes, the nostrils, and the lining of internal organs, like your gut. An allergic reaction can strike at any of these points.

The job of the immune system is to protect the body from toxins and pathogens that could cause disease. Your immune cells are supposed to distinguish between benign substances and foreign substances that can do the body significant harm. In the case of allergy, your immune cells get confused.

When your immune cells are exposed to a foreign substance, called an antigen, such as a bacterium or virus, they produce specific proteins called antibodies (or immunoglobulins), which tag the protein so that other immune cells know that they should attack it. Once an antibody is produced against a particular antigen, the immune cells are forever on guard against that antigen. The next time you are exposed to that antigen, your body will attack it. That's why once you get chicken pox or measles you don't get it again, because your body is ready to pounce the minute it reappears.

The antibody/antigen response works really well when dealing with real enemies, like the chicken pox virus, but if you're allergic, it works against you. In the case of allergy, your immune cells produce antibodies against substances that mean you no harm. In fact, it's your body's reaction to the substance that is causing you trouble, not the substance itself. For example, if you're allergic to pollen, every time you are exposed to pollen, your immune system begins producing a particular antibody called IgE, which is involved in all allergic reactions. IgE stimulates special cells called *mast cells* to release *histamine,* a chemical that is important for digestion and the dilation of small blood vessels, but that in excess can cause allergic symptoms. The release of histamine is what causes your runny nose, itchy, watery eyes, and general feelings of misery (it also stimulates pain receptors). But your allergic reaction doesn't end there. During an allergic attack, your immune system revs up production of other cells called leukotrienes and prostaglandins and other allergy mediators, which cause inflammation. Constant exposure to inflammation can cause damage to healthy tissues and organs, and in fact, can do particular harm to your lungs in the case of asthma. To add to your woes, inflammation promotes the formation of troublesome chemicals in the body called free radicals, which can cause further damage throughout your body.

Although we often say allergy and asthma in the same breath, they are not the same problem. Although it may be triggered by an allergy, asthma is a chronic inflammatory condition of the respiratory system. It is characterized by obstructed airways caused when bronchial tubes become inflamed, constricted, and clogged with mucus. During an asthma attack, the airways can become so constricted that the sufferer is literally gasping for breath. Although it can be managed successfully, asthma can be life-threatening, and medical attention is always required. As noted earlier, an asthma attack can be caused by an allergen, like pollen, or it can be triggered by exercise, cold air, or chemicals such as cigarette smoke or pollution, or by an allergic reaction to a food additive.

WHAT ALLERGY IS *NOT*

There's another misconception about allergy that I would like to clear up—an allergy is not an intolerance. For example, millions of people, myself included, cannot tolerate dairy products because we lack an enzyme to digest it properly. The condition is called lactose intolerance. Millions more can't eat grains because they cannot digest a protein in most grains called gluten—the condition is called gluten intolerance. Although the symptoms may be similar, neither of these problems is a true allergy. In reality, an allergy is a very specific immune reaction involving production of the IgE antibody.

Although most allergies are not life-threatening, allergy is not a trivial problem. First and foremost, allergies can make people miserable. In fact, allergic symptoms account for 3.8 million missed work and school days each year. And allergies exact a steep financial toll on the economy. We spend $4.5 billion annually in doctors' visits and medication. In addition, allergies may threaten our health in ways that are not quite fully understood. For example, some studies suggest that unrecognized food allergies may be linked to numerous medical conditions such as Chronic Obstructive Pulmonary Disease (chronic bronchitis and emphysema), rheumatoid arthritis, an autoimmune disease in which the body's immune cells attack the joints, Attention Deficit Disorder in children, and even migraine headaches. Allergic rhinitis (a fancy name for the stuffy, itchy nose caused by hay fever) is a leading cause of recurrent sinusitis or sinus infections, an inflammation of the sinus membranes that plagues tens of millions of people and often leads to sinus surgery, which often doesn't solve the problem. I'm not telling you this to scare you, but to show you why it's important to get your allergies under control.

WHY THE INCREASE IN ALLERGY?

Although there is no doubt that the incidence of allergy is increasing dramatically, the nature of allergies remains a medical mystery. No one knows why some people get allergies and other people don't. Genetics clearly plays a role. Some allergies, especially food allergies, tend to run in families. If you have one allergic parent, you stand a 20 to 50 percent chance of developing an allergy, but not necessarily the same allergy as your parent. If you have two allergic parents, there's up to a 75 percent chance that you too will be allergic to something.

Genetics alone, however, cannot explain the rapid and unprecedented increase in allergy over the past hundred years. Our genes haven't changed, yet our susceptibility to allergy has increased. Scientists blame the allergy epidemic on everything from changing weather trends due to global warming, which increases exposure to pollen, to air pollution, which weakens the respiratory system, to the dumping of thousands of chemical additives into the food supply, which poses a serious challenge to the immune system. The true cause of the increase in allergy is probably a combination of several factors.

Increased exposure to chemicals is high on my list of probable culprits. The amount of new chemicals introduced into the environment is mind boggling. According to the U.S. Environmental Protection Agency, in just one year (1994), more than 2.2 billion pounds of toxic chemicals were released into the environment in the United States. What happens when those chemicals enter our bodies? The body has an elaborate system to detoxify dangerous chemicals, but the body can become overwhelmed, which will have a negative impact on every system, including the immune system. In fact, some scientists speculate that the constant exposure to toxins can shift the immune system into overdrive, triggering allergic reactions and autoimmune diseases.

Moreover, because a disproportionate number of affluent people suffer from allergies, many researchers believe that the same practices that have dramatically extended life span, such as improved hygiene and childhood vaccinations, may inadvertently have disrupted normal immune function so that immune cells overreact to normally harmless substances.

Overexposure to antibiotics is another potential allergy trigger. If overused, antibiotics may harm immune function, interfering with the ability of immune cells to communicate with each other, which can lead to the kind of confusion that results in cells attacking harmless substances. In addition, antibiotics not only kill bad bacteria, they kill good bacteria that live in the intestines and help to normalize immune function. Many studies have shown that people with autoimmune diseases (in which the immune system mistakenly attacks the tissues of the body) typically have low levels of good bacteria in their gut.

ALLERGY TREATMENTS

The allergy epidemic has spawned a multi-billion-dollar industry consisting of drugs, supplements, and other cutting-edge products designed to control allergy symptoms. The standard treatments for allergy—allergy shots and antihistamine medications and nasal sprays—do work, but only up to a point. As any allergy sufferer knows, these treatments have their downside. First, many commonly used antihistamines can have nasty side effects such as dry mouth and heart palpitations, and may not be safe for people with heart disease, high blood pressure, or diabetes. The primary problem with antihistamines, however, is that they make users sleepy and less alert. In fact, a recent study reported in *Annals of Internal Medicine* noted that one common over-the-counter antihistamine, Benadryl, so seriously impaired the ability of drivers to operate a car that the drivers might as well have been driving drunk. Although the newest generation of allergy drugs, such as Claritin and Allegra, are less likely to cause drowsiness, they are expensive, are not covered by many health plans, and have side effects—such as dizziness and sleep disorders—of their own.

Allergy shots or immunotherapy work well for many but not all people. Allergy shots are given primarily for airborne allergies, such as pollen. Each treatment entails injecting a tiny amount of the allergen under the skin—not enough to cause an allergic response, but enough to alert the immune system that something new is being introduced into the body. Eventually, over time, the body should become desensitized to the allergen so that it no longer responds by attacking it. Allergy shots have their downside, though. They are expensive and inconvenient, because they must be administered by a doctor and may require several years to take full effect.

Asthma and severe allergies are often treated with steroids in the form of inhalers or nose sprays, and are sometimes even taken internally in serious cases. Although they are great at relieving symptoms, at least for a while, long-term use of steroids can have particularly nasty side effects, including dampened immune function, which increases your susceptibility to infection, thinning bones, and even memory loss.

My problem with all of these conventional therapies is that they are all geared to treating symptoms, but they do not get to the underlying problem causing the allergy in the first place. The natural approach in treating allergy and asthma is different and, in my experience, more effective in the long run. Although we recognize that controlling symptoms is important, we also feel that it is of equal importance to create an environment in the body that makes it allergy resistant. By that I mean that our goal is to relieve symptoms and reduce exposure to toxins that weaken immune function while at the same time bolstering the immune system so that it is less likely to succumb to allergy.

I'm not saying that you should throw away your medicine, not at all! But it is my hope that in time, you will need to use it less and less, and that eventually, you will be able to control your symptoms with simple, natural therapies that do not have side effects and, in fact, often have many other benefits in addition to controlling allergy. (For a more complete description of the pharmaceutical drugs used to treat allergy and asthma, turn to Chapter 12.)

THE ALTERNATIVES

More and more, allergy sufferers are rejecting the notion that they must take strong drugs to control their symptoms and are turning to alternative methods to treat and, more important, *prevent* their symptoms. They are spending millions of dollars on antiallergy supplements, including herbal remedies such as quercetin, stinging nettles, and MSM. These supplements do not have the same nasty side effects as conventional drugs, yet they are surprisingly effective. In Chapter 3, you will find my list of the Hot 55 Antiallergy Supplements with information on how to use them.

Allergy sufferers are also investing in household products such as high-tech vacuum cleaners, air purifiers, antiallergy laundry detergents, and bedding designed to "allergy proof" their homes, their workplaces, and even their cars! They are turning to drug-free treatments, such as acupuncture, hypnosis, homeopathy, and other forms of alternative therapy. Unfortunately, for most people, finding the right alternative allergy treatment is a hit or miss proposition. There are few sources of solid information about which of these products and treatments actually work and which are just a waste of money. Nor do people fully understand how to use these products effectively. In the pages of this book, you will find the answers to your questions about allergy control products and other alternative remedies. You will learn about the best methods of controlling your indoor allergies, outdoor allergies, food allergies, and skin allergies.

My goal is to empower you with the solid, up-to-date, scientifically based information you need to successfully manage your allergy symptoms on their own, or enhance the treatment you are receiving from doctors.

As every allergy sufferer knows, allergy can have a significant impact on your lifestyle. It can limit your activities outdoors, make you cautious about eating out, and even make you think twice about visiting friends and family. In some cases, it can even limit your choice of occupation. I am writing this book to help allergy sufferers live as full and unrestricted lives as possible, and to be as drug-free as possible.

Should You Be Tested?

You sneeze every time you're near a cat; your throat gets itchy after you eat a peanut; or your eyes start to tear every May at the start of hay fever season. Sometimes figuring out whether you are allergic to something is a "no brainer," but sometimes, it can be trickier. You may have symptoms but not know the cause, especially if you're allergic to something like dust mites (microscopic bugs in dust) and mold, which can strike at any time of the year.

If you have allergic symptoms, talk to your doctor or natural healer. Your M.D. may refer you to an allergist, a board-certified specialist in the treatment of allergy. If you go this route, I recommend that you see someone who is nutritionally oriented, and who is willing to incorporate treatments other than drugs into your therapy. Some people may choose to be treated by a naturopathic physician (ND) who is trained in both conventional and alternative therapies. Some of you may be fortunate enough to be seeing a complementary physician, an M.D. who uses both conventional and alternative therapies when appropriate.

Simply by taking a good medical history, you and your doctor may get to the root of the problem. For example, if your symptoms get worse on weekends after an afternoon of gardening, it's pretty obvious that you probably have a pollen allergy. If your symptoms get worse in the winter, it's a good sign that you may have a dust and mold allergy.

Depending on the severity of your symptoms, you may need to identify the precise problem so that you can treat it. If you're just using general allergy medication (such as an antihistamine or a decongestant) it's less important to know the precise allergen, but if you're going to undergo immunotherapy (allergy shots), your doctor needs to know the exact antigen.

Some allergies, especially food allergies, can be life-threatening. Therefore, if you have a potentially serious food allergy—for example, if you're allergic to peanuts or dairy products—you may need to go to great lengths to avoid these foods. You may not even be able to be in the same room with people eating them! But before you turn your life upside down to accommodate an allergy, you should know for sure that it's absolutely necessary.

Allergy testing can provide some concrete answers. There are two kinds of allergy tests that are performed at a doctor's office—the skin test and the blood test. Most allergists use a simple skin test to determine if you are allergic. A diluted extract of the allergen (pollen, dust mite, mold, or food) is either applied to a tiny scratch on your skin (the prick test) or injected into the top layer of skin (the intracutaneous test), usually on the back or arm. If you are allergic to the substance, the area exposed to the allergen will become red and irritated, forming a welt or wheal. Irritation is a sign that your body has produced IgE antibody to the antigen, but it doesn't necessarily mean that the particular substance is causing your problem. The downside of skin testing is that if you are highly allergic to a substance, if you are exposed to even a minute quantity of it, in rare cases, it could trigger anaphylactic shock and even death. This is particularly true for food allergies. Although this is rare, it is a risk. Also, if you are prone to eczema and other skin rashes, the test results may not be as accurate because your skin is easily irritated.

Blood testing (known as radioallergosorbent test or RAST) is another option. A blood sample is taken from the patient and checked for IgE antibodies to the particular antigen. It is not as accurate as skin testing, but it poses no risk because the patient is never directly exposed to the antigen.

Not everyone needs to undergo allergy testing. If your symptoms are mild and consistent, and you're pretty certain what's causing them, you can begin an allergy desensitization program on your own, that is, avoid the allergy and take steps to allergy proof your home or work area. If you have severe and chronic symptoms and you're not sure what's causing them, I think it's a good idea to undergo the appropriate allergy testing. However, I recommend that you see a nutritionally oriented physician who is willing to explore all treatment options, not just one who writes a prescription and sends you on your way.

The third kind of allergy test—the food elimination test—may be performed at home in most cases. If you suspect that a particular food is causing your problem, you eliminate it from your diet for a few days, then reintroduce it and see if your symptoms return. Proceed with caution! *This test is not a good idea for people with severe allergies because of the risk of anaphylactic shock.* In fact, in some cases, this test may be performed in a hospital should the patient require immediate care.

Is It a Cold or an Allergy?

Only time will tell! At least at first, it can be very difficult to distinguish between a cold and an allergy. Although both begin with an itchy, runny nose and even a scratchy throat, they don't end up the same way, and here are some tips on how to tell the two apart.

Check your tissues! If you have an allergy, your nasal secretions are thin and clear. If you have a cold, your nasal secretions are thicker, and may change color to green or yellow, signifying an infection.

A true cold should last between seven and ten days, with symptoms improving by around day five or so. An allergy can go on indefinitely, with no improvement.

If you have low-grade fever, you probably have a cold.

If you seem to develop a cold during the same time each year, it could be a sign of a seasonal allergy.

If you have a seasonal allergy, your symptoms will get worse outdoors.

Even if it's not hay fever season, you could still be having an allergic reaction to an indoor allergen, such as dust, mold, or a pet.

If symptoms do not end after two weeks, and you're still miserable, whether you have a cold or an allergy, check with your physician. (Of course, if you suddenly feel very sick or spike a high fever, call your M.D. immediately.)

Allergy testing can determine whether you have an allergy, and what you are allergic to.

Laughter: The Best Medicine?

Are your allergies acting up? According to a Japanese researcher, a good laugh may be just what the doctor ordered! A Kyoto allergist studied twenty-six people with atopic dermatitis, or skin hives triggered by allergens such as pet dander, dust, and pollen. After seeing a video of *Modern Times,* a hilarious film starring Charlie Chaplin, patients experienced significantly less allergic response on a standard skin test than before watching the movie. Why? The researcher speculates that laughter is a great stress reliever, and it is well known that stress can alter normal immune function. This is one treatment that is absolutely safe for everyone, and there no negative side effects. See if it works for you!

Are We Too Clean?

It's called the Hygiene Hypothesis. Some scientists believe that the exponential increase in the incidence of allergy in the past century is due in part to our obsession with cleanliness! Here's why. Before the twentieth century, when most people lived on farms or in rural settings, toddlers used to crawl around on dirt floors or in backyards that were teeming with microorganisms, in sharp contrast to the antiseptic, scrubbed-down nurseries of today.

Although the mere thought of babies eating dirt would send most modern parents into a tizzy, the fact is, many researchers believe that dirt contains beneficial bacteria that are meant to work in synergy with the immune system. In addition, the early and chronic exposure to both friendly and unfriendly bacteria taught young immune systems how to distinguish between friend and foe. Since young immune systems can no longer learn these valuable lessons from firsthand experience, they are not as able to differentiate between the good guys and the bad guys and become allergy prone. (I'm not suggesting that we feed babies dirt—there are cleaner ways of restoring good bacteria in our bodies. See Probiotics on page 95.)

We compound this problem by giving young children antibiotics, especially when they don't really need them. Antibiotics not only kill off both good and bad bacteria, but if given too often, may hamper normal immune function.

Some critics of modern medicine contend that childhood vaccinations against diseases such as measles, mumps, whooping cough, and chicken pox are also responsible for the increase in allergy. They claim that by vaccinating children, we are denying their immune systems the experience of battling illness and are creating "bored" immune cells that later attack nonthreatening substances. In addition, vaccinations may overstimulate particular immune cells responsible for allergy. This is a hotly debated topic among scientists, but the fact of the matter is, before vaccinations, death from childhood diseases was commonplace. Today, it is rare for children to die in infancy or early childhood. To me, if the price of preventing a crippling disease such as polio is hay fever later in life, so be it!

Concerned parents can protect their children against too much modern interference by giving them antibiotics only when absolutely necessary, and by not routinely using antibacterial products, such as soaps or cleaning supplies, in their homes. These products were meant to be used in hospitals to protect workers against serious infections like staph, not for casual use. The overuse of these products may in the long run have a harmful effect on immune function, contributing to problems such as allergy and autoimmune disease. Nor will these products keep us safe from infectious disease. Ironically, the more these products are used, the greater the risk of developing antibiotic-resistant infections that can be life-threatening.

CHAPTER 2

A Guide to Antiallergy Supplements

OUT OF THE HUNDREDS OF SUPPLEMENTS ON THE MAR-ket, I have picked the Hot 55 Antiallergy Supplements, which I consider to be the most helpful for people with allergic conditions. I am not suggesting that everyone should take all fifty-*five!* Some of you may do well taking a select few, others may find that your symptoms are best controlled when you take a combination formula containing up to a dozen or so supplements. Regardless of how many supplements you take, I feel that it's critical that you understand what you are taking, how to take it correctly, and why you are taking it. In my experience, if you don't know why you're doing what you are doing, you are less likely to be vigilant about taking your supplements.

Unlike conventional medicine, the natural approach to allergy control is to tackle the underlying cause of the problem, not simply to mask the symptoms with a strong drug. As you read over the description of each of the top antiallergy supplements, you will see the ingenious way in which supplements work. Many supplements have a direct effect on allergic symptoms, and are kinder and gentler versions of the antihistamines sold over the counter and by prescription. Very often, they have far fewer side effects than stronger drugs. But the power of the antiallergy supplements goes way beyond symptom relief—*they are powerful health enhancers.* For example, many supplements are antioxidants, which are natural compounds that protect us from free radicals, chemicals produced by the body as a by-product of energy production that can aggravate allergy and asthma. In fact, high levels of free radicals and low levels of antioxidants are common among asthmatics as well as people with other chronic illnesses. Other supplements have natural anti-inflammatory action. Inflammation, a by-product of allergy, can not only worsen your symptoms, but can be very harmful to your lungs and other organ systems of the body. Still other supplements normalize immune function, making it less likely that you will develop allergies in the first place.

And the best part is, unlike drugs that have endless negative side effects, most of the supplements I have selected have significant positive side *benefits.* They are not only good for allergy control, but many also help protect against other common diseases, such as heart disease, cancer, and arthritis.

In the section below, I will answer some basic questions about the Hot 55 Antiallergy Supplements so that you can become a knowledgeable supplement consumer.

What is a nutritional supplement?

A nutritional supplement is a nonfood nutrient used to enhance health. It is not a substitute for a good diet, but it can help fill in the gaps if you are not eating as carefully as you should. There are several different categories of supplements, including vitamins, minerals, herbs, herbal extracts (chemical compounds derived from herbs), phytochemicals, enzymes, and amino acids. Individual supplements can be sold separately, or can be combined in formulas designed to treat specific medical needs, such as formulas to relieve allergy symptoms, strengthen immune function, or improve joint health.

A *vitamin* is an organic substance necessary for life that is not produced by the body and must be obtained through food or supplements. There are two kinds of vitamins, water-soluble and fat-soluble. Water-soluble vitamins (such as vitamin C and the B vitamins) are not stored in the body and excess intake is excreted in urine. Water-soluble vitamins are measured in micrograms (mcg) or milligrams (mg). Fat-soluble vitamins (A, D, E, and K) are stored in fat deposits in the body. They are measured in IU, international units, with the exception of vitamin A, which is sometimes measured in RE, retinol units.

A *mineral* is a naturally occurring element found in the body that must be replenished through food or supplements. There are two types of minerals, trace minerals (you only need a minuscule quantity to survive) and essential minerals (you may need several grams a day). Trace minerals are measured in mcg, essential minerals are measured in mg or grams.

An *herb* refers to any plant or plant part (stem, leaf, fruit, root) that is used for its medicinal qualities. Although many natural food stores still sell loose, dried herbs that can be brewed into tea, in most cases, herbs are now sold in capsules, pills, and easy-to-use liquids. Most herbs contain one or more active ingredients that are responsible for their beneficial effects. In many cases, these ingredients are now sold separately as supplements in their own right. Like vitamins and minerals, herbs are measured in mcg, mg, or grams. In some cases, however, you may be instructed to take one or two capsules as opposed to a specific amount. Why? Herbal medicine is an ancient tradition dating back thousands of years. Although in recent years there have been many studies validating the science behind herbs, the fact is, herbal medicine is not an exact science. The dosing of herbs is often not as precise as the dosing of vitamins and minerals. This isn't surprising—in the old days, herbalists used to prescribe a cup of tea, or a few ounces of extract derived from a cooked root. They did not dose to the nearest mg, nor they did they need to. Most (certainly not all!) herbs are benign substances, and taking a bit more than you need is not going to harm you. In many cases, since the content of the active ingredients in plants vary from soil to soil, it was impossible to predict the precise amount of herb needed for the desired effect. Thanks to scientific methods, today, it is possible to buy standardized herbs with guaranteed potency, meaning you are getting enough of the active ingredient in the plant to be helpful.

Phytochemicals are chemicals derived from plants (fruits, vegetables, legumes, and grains) that have health benefits. Many phytochemicals have been isolated from plants and are sold as supplements.

Enzymes are proteins that bring about chemical changes; *coenzymes* are proteins that work with enzymes. They are both produced by the body and found in food.

Amino acids are the building blocks of protein. Nonessential amino acids are produced by the body; essential amino acids must be obtained through food. In recent years, we have learned that specific amino acids have powerful health benefits if taken at doses higher than what is normally found in food, and therefore, may need to be supplemented.

Herbal Power

Between 25 and 50 percent of the drugs on the market today either are derived from plant sources or contain chemical imitations of plant compounds. The chemicals ephedrine and pseudoephedrine, found in many over-the-counter cold and allergy remedies, are derived from the ephedra plant. The asthma drug Cromolyn was derived from chromones, a natural bronchodilator extracted from the khella plant (*Ammi visnaga*), native to the Middle East.

Can I be allergic to some supplements?

Absolutely! For example, if you have a pollen allergy, some herbal supplements, such as chamomile or echinacea, may trigger an allergic response. In fact, if you are highly allergic to many plants, I strongly advise you to steer clear of botanical-based supplements—that is, supplements derived from herbs. There are numerous others to choose from. I am not suggesting that every allergic person avoid all herbal supplements. In fact, one of the most successful treatments for hay fever is a plant—stinging nettles. It has been shown to relieve allergic symptoms for many people. If, however, you can't look at a plant without feeling your eyes tear and your chest tighten, definitely steer clear of botanicals.

You can also be allergic to an additive in a supplement, just as you can be allergic to an additive in a pharmaceutical drug. For example, you can't be allergic to vitamins, because you could not survive without them, but it's possible to be allergic to the soy oil used in your vitamin pill, or the cornstarch or dairy by-products used as fillers and binders. Therefore, you must read the label carefully before buying any product. Look for products that do not contain artificial flavoring, and if you are allergic to either corn, soy, dairy, yeast, wheat, or gluten, be sure to buy products that specifically state that they do not have these ingredients. If in doubt, call the manufacturer to be sure. IF YOU ARE HIGHLY ALLERGIC TO A SUBSTANCE, EVEN A SMALL AMOUNT OF IT CAN TRIGGER SYMPTOMS.

Can I take supplements with prescription medication?

If you are not taking any medication, you can try using supplements alone and see if you get enough allergy relief. Many of you will find that your supplement regimen will reduce, if not eliminate, symptoms of seasonal allergies and will reduce chronic allergic symptoms. If you are taking prescription medication, in most cases, you can take your supplements along with prescription allergy or asthma medication. However, you should consult your doctor before taking any natural supplements that may interact with your medication. Over time, as the supplements take effect, you may need less "rescue" medication. Tell your doctor what supplements you are taking, par-

ticularly if you are being treated for other health problems
or are undergoing any medical procedures. Some supplements are natural blood thinners, which is good because
they prevent blood clots, but may interfere with healing
after surgery. In addition, some supplements may interact
with your prescription medication. If your physician is
clueless about supplements, ask your pharmacist to check
whether there is a risk of interaction. Many pharmacists
are surprisingly knowledgeable about both medication
and supplements, because most dispense both. (And I'm
not just saying this because I'm a pharmacist!)

How are supplements sold?

Supplements are sold in many different forms. Most of
the supplements that I recommend come in convenient
capsules, pills, or tablets. Others are sold as powders that
must be taken with liquid, liquid extracts, and teas. Although each supplement is available separately, in recent
years, there has been a trend to combine supplements in
special formulas designed to treat a specific problem. For
example, if you go to your natural food store or pharmacy,
you will see row upon row of antiallergy formulas containing up to a dozen or even more individual herbs, vitamins, or phytochemicals. In all likelihood, you will find
nearly all of the ingredients listed in the Hot 55.

*Which brands of supplements are the best, and where
is the best place to buy them?*

Supplements are sold everywhere today, from the Internet to natural food stores to discount pharmacies and even
supermarkets. Choose the location that is most convenient
for you and offers the best selection of products. There are

numerous brands on the market, some better than others. Stick to reputable brands and don't be swayed by the cheapest price. There is a wide variation in quality, and in many cases, you get what you pay for. If possible, try to purchase products that are labeled pharmaceutical grade, which means they are of the highest quality and free of impurities. You may not be able to tell a lot about a book from its cover, but you can tell a lot about a supplement by its packaging. A careful manufacturer will offer its product in a tamper-proof, sealed container. The product should have an easy-to-read label containing all the ingredients. Each product should have an expiration date and a lot number so that if there is any problem, the manufacturer can quickly pull the affected product off the shelves.

I recommend that you purchase herbal supplements that are organically grown, and are devoid of pesticides, artificial color, or other chemical additives.

To maintain potency, supplements should be stored in a cool, dark place out of direct sunlight. Some supplements, however, need to be refrigerated. Check the label for information on storage and handling.

When should I take my supplements?

The rule of thumb is, most supplements are best absorbed when taken with food. It is also less likely that a supplement will cause stomach upset if taken with a full stomach. On rare occasions, I will tell you to take a specific supplement between meals because it is one that is best absorbed on an empty stomach.

How long will I have to take supplements before I see any results?

Please keep in mind that supplements rarely work overnight. In most cases, it can take two to four weeks for the full effect to kick in. If you have seasonal allergies, it's best to begin taking your antiallergy regimen at least one month before your symptoms usually kick in. If you have year-round allergies, you should take your supplements every day. Sometimes, your supplement regimen may work very well for a while, and then your symptoms may return. If this happens, you should switch to a different regimen.

Are any supplements dangerous?

As I have been telling people for decades, that a substance purports to be "natural" doesn't mean it's safe. Some manufacturers are not as honest as others, and are selling products that have dubious safety records. In some cases, a product that is used correctly may be safe for most people, but has the potential to be abused, as in the case of ephedra, a time-honored herbal cold and allergy treatment that has been badly misused, and therefore, has gotten a bad rap. (Ephedra should not be used by people with heart problems or high blood pressure. For more information, see page 56.) The supplements that I describe in the Hot 55 are safe for most people, but when they are not, I caution specific readers not to use them. Pregnant women and nursing mothers and people with pre-existing medical conditions should be especially careful about using either drugs or supplements without first checking with their physicians or natural healers.

Of all the supplements listed, how do I know which will work for me?

As you read over the Hot 55 Antiallergy Supplements, you find that each supplement offers its own unique benefits, and some may seem more appropriate for your particular allergies than others. For example, if you find that your allergies are often triggered by infection, you may want to read up on supplements that boost and normalize immune function. If you feel that you're not getting enough antioxidants in your diet, you will want to see which antioxidants you should be taking. If you have asthma, you will be interested to read about the select group of supplements that may help control your symptoms. If you suffer from eczema or psoriasis, two skin conditions associated with allergy, you may want to try some supplements that may help improve your skin. If you have arthritis, you may want to take an antiallergy supplement that can also relieve the pain and inflammation in your joints. After reading over the Hot 55, you may decide to try to take one or two antiallergy supplements, or go for a more comprehensive combination formula. You may try one regimen for a few weeks, then include more supplements to see if you can get even better symptom relief. I have provided you with the information, but I understand that everybody is different, and that when it comes to allergy control, one size does not fit all. Therefore, please use this information to devise the program that works best for you.

Earl Mindell's Hot 55
Antiallergy Supplements

1. Vitamin A	29. Green tea
2. Vitamin B-complex	30. Gumweed
3. Boswellia	31. Histidine
4. Bromelain	32. Horseradish
5. Butterbur	33. Jewelweed
6. Vitamin C	34. Licorice
7. Cayenne	35. Lobelia
8. Chinese skullcap	36. Lungwort
9. Coenzyme Q10 (Co Q10)	37. Magnesium
	38. Marshmallow
10. Colostrum	39. Milk thistle
11. Curcumin	40. MSM (methyl sulfonyl methane)
12. Digestive enzymes	
13. Dong quai	41. Mullein
14. Vitamin E	42. NAC (N-acetyl cysteine)
15. Elderberry	
16. Elecampane	43. Perilla oil
17. Ephedra	44. Probiotics
18. Essential fatty acids	45. Quercetin
19. Eucalyptus	46. Reishi mushroom
20. Eyebright	47. Sarsaparilla
21. Fenugreek	48. Selenium
22. Feverfew	49. Stinging nettles
23. Flavonoids	50. Synephrine
24. Forskolin	51. Thyme
25. Garlic	52. Tylophora
26. Ginger root	53. Wild cherry
27. Gingko	54. Yerba santa
28. Grape seed extract	55. Zinc

CHAPTER 3

The Hot 55 Antiallergy Supplements

VITAMIN A

When you think of Vitamin A, you probably think of healthy skin and good vision. What you may not know is that A could also stand for "allergy fighter." Vitamin A helps protect and soothe the lungs and mucous membranes, which are likely to be irritated by airborne allergies. In fact, people with asthma typically have lower-than-normal levels of vitamin A in their lungs, which means that they may be using it up faster. Vitamin A is also an immune booster, which enhances the body's ability to fight infection. The last thing you need on top of your allergies is a nasty cold! Another benefit is that it's an antioxidant, which protects the body against damage by highly reactive oxygen molecules called free radicals.

There are two types of vitamin A: preformed vitamin A and provitamin A, better known as beta carotene. Preformed vitamin A is found in animal products such as milk, eggs, and liver. Beta carotene is found in fruits and vegetables and is converted into vitamin A in the body. I personally prefer beta carotene over preformed vitamin A because I think it's safer. Why not just take vitamin A? Vitamin A is a fat-soluble vitamin, which means that it can be stored in fat. Therefore, it's possible to accumulate too much vitamin A, which can be toxic. However, the body will only make as much vitamin A from beta carotene as it needs, and discard the rest, so there is no danger of toxicity with beta carotene.

Vitamin A is not for everyone. In excess, it may cause birth defects, which is why both vitamin A and beta carotene supplements should be avoided by pregnant women unless prescribed by their physicians. Smokers beware—avoid products that contain either beta carotene or vitamin A. In a major Finnish study, smokers who took either beta carotene or 25,000 IU of vitamin A daily had a higher death rate from lung cancer than smokers who did not! What's odd about this result is that people who eat foods rich in beta carotene (yellow and orange fruits and vegetables) have substantially *lower* rates of cancer than those who do not. No one knows why beta carotene or vitamin A supplementation would increase lung cancer rates, but scientists speculate that chemicals in smoke may alter beta carotene, and vitamin A, in unhealthy ways. Of course, the best advice is to quit smoking, which only aggravates allergies anyway.

Possible Benefits

Protects delicate mucous membranes.
Boosts and normalizes immune function.
Antioxidant.

How to Use It

Take one (5,000 IU) capsule of vitamin A daily, or one (10,000–15,000 IU) capsule of beta carotene daily. Check your multivitamin—you may already be getting enough vitamin A or beta carotene. Vitamin A is also included in many antiallergy combination formulas, so be sure to read the label carefully to make sure that you are taking the right amount.

VITAMIN B-COMPLEX

If you suffer from allergy symptoms, be sure to take a supplement containing the full range of vitamin Bs. Vitamin B is also an immune booster, which enhances the body's ability to fight infection. The last thing you need on top of your allergies is a nasty cold! Another benefit is that it's an antioxidant, which protects your body against damage by highly reactive oxygen molecules called free radicals. I know that B vitamins are also sold individually, but as a rule, they are meant to work together in the body, which is why I advise people to take B-complex as opposed to individual B vitamins. (In some cases, however, you may need to take a bit more of one B vitamin than is in the standard B-complex combination, as you will see.) The Bs are essential for a wide range of bodily functions, including the production of protective antioxidants, which help relieve allergy symptoms and normalize immune function. In addition, B-complex helps your body better cope with both physical and mental stress and enhances energy production by your cells. You know how dragged-out and tired you can feel during allergy season! Believe me, you'll feel worse if you don't get enough of your full range of vitamin Bs.

One B vitamin in particular, pantothenic acid, or vitamin B5, is particularly helpful for relieving the stuffy nose and congestion caused by hay fever and is often included in combination formulas to treat allergy. In fact, in one clinical study, patients taking two (250 mg) tablets of pantothenic acid reported a reduction in nasal allergy symptoms. Pantothenic acid is found in foods such as liver, yeast, salmon, and some fruits and vegetables, but it is also made in the gut by good bacteria. If you have been taking antibiotics, however, which can kill both good and bad bacteria, you may deplete your supply of this B vitamin. If you take a B-complex supplement, be sure it contains enough pantothenic acid, or you may need to take an additional amount, especially if you tend to feel depleted and stressed-out by your allergies. Pantothenic acid may also help reduce the occurrence of migraines, which may be aggravated by allergies.

Vitamin B12, cobalamin, can block an allergic response to sulfites, a common allergy in children. Sulfites are common preservatives used in dried fruits, wine, and other foods that can trigger bronchial spasm (asthma attacks) in susceptible people. (If you're allergic to sulfites, don't eat them.)

Possible Benefits

Helps you better cope with stress.
Reduces nasal congestion and allergy symptoms.

How to Use It

For B-complex, look for a formula that contains 25–50 mg of each of the B vitamins, including B1, thiamin; B2, riboflavin; B3, niacin; B5, pantothenic acid; B6, pyridoxine; and B12, cobalamin. Take one tablet daily. Please note that most multivitamins contain an adequate amount of B-complex, so if you are taking a multivitamin, you will not need to supplement.

For pantothenic acid, the usual dose for allergies is one (500 mg) tablet twice daily.

BOSWELLIA

Boswellia (Boswellia serrata) is a staple of the Ayurvedic traditional herbal medicine of India. In the United States, boswellia is best known as a treatment for rheumatoid arthritis, but it is also included in many combination herbal formulas to treat allergy. Why? Compounds derived from boswellia, boswellic acids, block the production of enzymes in the body that not only promote inflammation in the joints, but can irritate the bronchial tubes and stimulate excess mucus secretion. Inflammation not only destroys healthy tissues by itself, but also stimulates the production of free radicals, which inflict even more damage. Any inflammation that targets the respiratory system is at the very least going to worsen allergy symptoms, and at the very worst, may even trigger them. Some researchers believe that these same inflammatory enzymes may be involved in severe respiratory problems such as chronic bronchitis and cystic fibrosis.

Unlike standard nonsteroidal anti-inflammatory drugs (such as Advil and Motrin), boswellia does not irritate the stomach. In fact, natural healers prescribe it for ulcerative colitis, a condition that may be triggered by an allergic response in some people.

Here's another reason I think taking anti-inflammatory herbs like boswellia is especially important for people with allergies. In recent years, researchers have begun to take inflammation more seriously, and in fact, many believe that it is the root cause of nearly all disease, from cancer to heart disease to Alzheimer's. People with allergies are in a chronic state of inflammation; therefore, it is important to try to keep this potentially dangerous process under control.

Possible Benefits

Relieves inflammation.
May relieve chronic bronchitis.
Reduces mucus production.

How to Use It

Take three (500 mg) capsules or tablets daily until symptoms subside, then take one (500 mg) capsule or tablet daily. Or take a combination antiallergy formula including boswellia.

BROMELAIN

Bromelain is derived from a group of enzymes found in pineapple. Bromelain is widely touted as a digestive aid, a remedy for arthritis, and a natural wound healer. You may wonder how any one supplement can be so versatile. Bromelain's healing power stems from its anti-inflammatory action, and as discussed earlier, inflammation is involved in virtually every ailment known to man ranging from colds to cancer. Inflammation is also a nasty by-product of allergy and can contribute to the swelling of the nasal passages typical of sinusitis.

In one study of patients with sinusitis, bromelain was added as part of the treatment regimen in patients already taking antibiotics and antihistamines, the usual treatment for this condition. Those taking bromelain healed significantly faster (as measured by swelling of their nasal passages) than those who did not. Other studies have shown that bromelain may help thin out mucus secretions in the respiratory tract. Bromelain is not a stand-alone allergy remedy, rather it is often included in combination products containing quercetin, a rising star among flavonoids (see page 65), and vitamin C (see page 41). The bromelain-quercetin combo makes perfect sense. Although quercetin is a potent allergy fighter, like other flavonoids, it is not well absorbed by the body. On the other hand, bromelain is well absorbed and, in the process, enhances the absorption of other nutrients riding along on its coattails, including quercetin.

An added bonus: If you work out, bromelain may also help relieve those postexercise aches and pains.

Possible Benefits

Anti-inflammatory.
Enhances absorption of flavonoids.
Relieves sore, aching joints.

How to Use It

If using bromelain alone, take one (500 mg) capsule twice daily between meals.

If using bromelain with quercetin, take one (100 mg) capsule along with 400 mg quercetin (see page 97) up to three times daily with meals.

Personal Advice

Eating pineapple won't do it! Most of the enzymes used in bromelain are from the pineapple stem.

Caution

If you are allergic to pineapple, do not use bromelain.

BUTTERBUR

Can a little-known European herb be as effective a treatment for hay fever as a big-time pharmaceutical remedy? According to one Swiss study, the answer is a resounding Yes! Butterbur is an herb that grows in Europe, southwestern Asia, and northern Asia. For centuries, European healers have used the butterbur *(Petasites hybridus)* as a treatment for fever, headaches, and nearly everything else. Recently, a group of Swiss and German researchers compared the effectiveness of a standardized extract of butterbur against cetirizine, marketed as Zyrtec, a popular prescription allergy medicine. Out of 125 patients with hay fever, 61 were given butterbur and 64 were given cetirizine. After two weeks, patients in both groups were asked to assess their symptoms. Patients taking the butterbur extract and the cetirizine reported a similar reduction in symptoms, but those taking cetirizine experienced more drowsiness and fatigue. According to the Mindell rating system, the score is butterbur 1, cetirizine 0 (at least, according to this study). The researchers caution that more studies are needed before trading in your antihistamines for butterbur, but the early results are encouraging.

Migraine sufferers take note: Butterbur may help reduce the incidence and severity of your headaches.

Possible Benefits

Reduces hay fever symptoms.
Anti-inflammatory.
Helps prevent migraine headaches.

How to Use It

Take two (500 mg) capsules daily, or look for an antiallergy combination formula containing butterbur.

VITAMIN C

Thanks to my dear friend, the late Linus Pauling, Ph.D., vitamin C is best known as the supplement that can decrease the duration and intensity of the common cold. This is a considerable accomplishment considering that after decades of trying, the world's top pharmaceutical houses have been unable to invent a synthetic drug that works as well! This superstar among vitamins can also help relieve your allergy symptoms. Vitamin C is a natural antihistamine, which blocks the effect of histamine, the substance that causes the itchy, runny nose and watery eyes typical of an allergic reaction. Vitamin C is also an important antioxidant that helps control free radical attack in the body. In addition, in the body, vitamin C enhances the effectiveness of another important antioxidant, vitamin E. Several studies have shown that high doses of vitamin C (up to 2,000 mg daily) may also help asthmatics. Nearly two centuries ago, scientists noticed a link between scurvy, severe vitamin C deficiency, and asthma. More recently, researchers have found that there is an inverse relationship between vitamin C intake and asthma—that is, the rate of asthma *increases* as the intake of vitamin C in the diet *decreases*. Other studies have shown a low level of antioxidants such as vitamin C in the lung tissue of asthmatics, which is further depleted immediately following exposure to allergens, like pollen. If you find that your asthma is worse during allergy season, taking additional antioxidants, such as vitamin C, may help keep your symptoms at bay.

Robert Cathcart, M.D., a famous vitamin C researcher and physician, reported that ingesting very high levels of vitamin C, that is, to bowel tolerance (the point at which it produces an upset stomach and diarrhea), can dramatically reduce allergy and asthma symptoms, including those induced by food or drugs. Even at high doses, vitamin C is nontoxic. Since vitamin C is a water-soluble vitamin, what isn't absorbed by the body is eliminated in urine.

Vitamin C works in synergy with flavonoids (see page 65). In nature, you will find that foods that contain the highest levels of vitamin C (such as berries, red pepper, broccoli, and citrus fruits) also contain a hefty amount of flavonoids.

Vitamin C also helps control stress and can lessen the damaging effect of cortisol, which is pumped out by the adrenal glands when you're feeling tense or overwrought. As you may have noticed, your allergic symptoms tend to worsen when you're under stress, primarily because stress hormones can disrupt normal immune function and trigger an autoimmune response.

Possible Benefits

May relieve asthma symptoms, reduce incidence of asthma.

Antihistamine action reduces allergic response.

Normalizes immune function.

Strengthens immune system.

Important antioxidant.

How to Use It

Take one (500 mg) capsule or tablet three times daily. The ascorbate form contains a natural buffering agent that helps to prevent the stomach distress associated with high intake of vitamin C. Vitamin C works especially well with another Hot Antiallergy Supplement, MSM.

CAYENNE

Ever notice that when you eat a spicy meal, your nose begins to run and your sinuses are quickly cleared? So it shouldn't come as any surprise that cayenne *(Capsicum frutescens),* also known as red pepper, is being used in many antiallergy formulas. Cayenne helps thin out mucus secretions and is a good expectorant, which is helpful if your nasal passages are clogged during allergy season. Of course, you could get the same effect by eating a bowl of hot and sour soup, or a hot tamale!

Capsaicin, a substance in cayenne, is a natural anti-inflammatory.

Possible Benefits

Clears clogged sinuses.
Reduces pain and inflammation.

How to Use It

Cayenne is not a stand-alone allergy treatment, but may be included in combination antiallergy formulas to give them an added kick.

Caution

Do not use cayenne on a regular basis if you are taking an asthma medication with theophylline. Cayenne may increase its absorption, which can cause toxicity.

CHINESE SKULLCAP

The root of the Chinese skullcap plant (*Scutellaria baicalensis*) is frequently included in traditional Chinese medicine (TCM) antiallergy combination herbal formulas. It is a time-honored treatment for asthma. A member of the mint family, Chinese skullcap (different from American skullcap) is grown in China and Russia. Chinese skullcap is a natural antihistamine and is rich in flavonoids (see page 65). In fact, one particular flavonoid found in skullcap, baicalein, can inhibit the production of leukotrienes, inflammatory cells that cause the bronchial tubes to constrict, causing bronchial spasms. Chinese skullcap is a natural anti-inflammatory and has also been used to treat inflammatory skin conditions (such as psoriasis).

Like other Chinese herbs, Chinese skullcap is not meant to work alone; it works best when combined with other herbs.

Possible Benefits

Relieves asthma and allergy symptoms.
Reduces inflammation.

How to Use It

Look for an antiallergy combination formula containing Chinese skullcap. If you work with a Chinese healer, ask him or her for dried skullcap root to make into a tea.

COENZYME Q10 (CO Q10)

Co Q10 is a coenzyme, a substance that works with an enzyme (or protein) to bring about a chemical reaction within the body. Co Q10 is vital to the production of ATP, the cellular fuel that runs the body. In addition, it is a fat-soluble antioxidant that enhances the effect of another key antioxidant, vitamin E. Asthma and allergy sufferers typically have low levels of antioxidants, especially during allergy season. Like other antioxidants, Co Q10 helps control free radical activity, which can be caused by inflammation due to an allergic response. Taking Co Q10 alone will not defeat your allergies, but it works in synergy with other antiallergy supplements, which is why it is included in numerous antiallergy combination formulas.

There's another good reason to take Co Q10—it is great for your heart. In Japan and Italy, it used as a treatment for congestive heart failure. In the United States, innovative cardiologists are prescribing Co Q10 to their patients to prevent heart disease.

Possible Benefits

Strengthens antioxidant defenses in the body.

Can help increase energy production on the cellular level.

How to Use It

Take one (60 mg) capsule twice daily, or look for a multivitamin or antiallergy formula containing Co Q10.

COLOSTRUM

Colostrum is special fluid produced by nursing mammals only for the first forty-eight hours after giving birth. Bovine colostrum (a supplement derived from cows) has been touted as a panacea for nearly everything. It's been promoted as a performance booster for athletes, an anti-aging supplement for baby boomers, a natural fat burner, and an immune system regulator that helps to both fight disease and tone down an overactive immune system (as in the case of allergies). It's tempting to dismiss a "cure-all" as nothing but pure hype, but that's not the case with colostrum. There's some interesting science behind the claims that may be useful to allergy sufferers.

Colostrum contains special proteins that can help the immune system do a better job. For example, one type of protein, transfer factor, actually teaches the immature immune cells of a baby how to distinguish between friend and foe. An allergic reaction by definition is one in which the immune system overreacts to a normally harmless substance. Taking colostrum as an adult could possibly help "retrain" immune cells not to target benign substances, which could nip allergic reactions in the bud.

Another type of protein in colostrum, growth factors, helps the infant's digestive tract mature more quickly. As you know, infants can't eat real food because their gut is too "leaky," that is, foreign proteins that should stay in the gut are passed to the bloodstream where they can trigger a severe allergic reaction. That's why infants are only fed breast milk or formula. Growth factors help strengthen the gut, so that the infant can eventually eat real food. Many natural healers believe that some people develop "leaky gut" as adults, which may be at the root of their allergies. Taking colostrum with growth factors could help heal the gut, thereby preventing the foreign proteins from entering the system and causing an allergy attack.

Colostrum is particularly good for people who are chronically plagued with colds and sinusitis, and who can't ever seem to get well and stay well.

Possible Benefits

Normalizes an overactive immune system.
Protects against infection.

How to Use It

Take three (480 mg) capsules daily.

Caution

Colostrum is often touted as safe for people with milk allergies. However, if you are allergic to dairy products, I don't advise that you use this supplement. Better to be safe than sorry (and there are fifty-four others to choose from!).

CURCUMIN

Curcumin is an oil derived from the root of the turmeric plant *(Curcuma longa)*, a spice widely used in Indian cooking and a key component of curry powder. (It's the spice that gives curry its telltale yellow color.) Turmeric has been used for thousands of years in the Ayurvedic system of medicine to treat a wide range of ailments. Before the invention of refrigeration, turmeric and other spices were used to preserve food. We now know that these spices are potent antioxidants, which protect food from oxidation, or free radical attack, which can accelerate spoilage. We also know that the same mechanism occurs within our bodies, which is why antioxidant foods and supplements have become so popular.

Curcumin is included in many antiallergy formulas, often in combination with another herb, boswellia. In addition to its strong antioxidant action, curcumin is a powerful anti-inflammatory. In fact, studies of rheumatoid arthritis patients have shown that curcumin works as well in terms of reducing inflammation as well-known prescription drugs, but without the stomach upset typical of nonsteroidal anti-inflammatory medications. In a clinical study conducted in India, curcumin was used successfully to treat patients with chronic respiratory disorders, which can also be aggravated by inflammation.

Taking curcumin alone will probably not relieve your allergy symptoms, but will enhance the effect of other antiallergy supplements.

Possible Benefits

Antioxidant.

Anti-inflammatory.

Proven to relieve respiratory symptoms such as coughing and shortness of breath.

How to Use It

Look for an antiallergy combination formula containing curcumin.

Caution

Curcumin is a natural blood thinner. If you are taking other blood thinners, check with your doctor before using a supplement with curcumin.

Personal Advice

Curcumin can also lower high cholesterol levels, and preliminary studies suggest it may be a potent cancer fighter. You get so much more from using these "full-spectrum" natural healing agents than from simply popping an antihistamine!

DIGESTIVE ENZYMES

The major difference between the conventional and natural approaches to treating allergies is that conventional practitioners focus on symptom relief, whereas natural healers try to get to the root of the problem, that is, they try to find the underlying cause that is forcing the immune system to malfunction. The use of digestive enzymes to treat allergy is a prime example of what I mean. A growing number of natural healers and progressive physicians suspect that allergies may be triggered by partially digested proteins that pass through the gut into the bloodstream, causing confusion among immune cells, which attack it as a "foreign" protein. This condition is called Leaky Gut Syndrome. Chronically overstimulated immune cells then begin to attack other harmless proteins, resulting in allergies to food and other benign substances, such as pollen. Some healers also believe that the same scenario may be at the root of other autoimmune problems such as rheumatoid arthritis and multiple sclerosis.

Why do some people have difficulty digesting protein? They may not produce enough of the digestive enzymes needed to adequately break down protein. Digestive enzymes are produced by the pancreas and are also present in food. The body's production of digestive enzymes can be disrupted by any number of factors, including hormonal shifts, stress, poor nutrition, and aging. Low levels of the digestive enzymes can result in vitamin deficiencies, especially of the B vitamins, which are extremely important in helping the body withstand stress. The solution is to give supplements of digestive enzymes—proteases or proteolytic enzymes—to help the body better digest and absorb proteins. These enzymes include trypsin and chymotrypsin, which also have natural anti-inflammatory action. A good digestive enzyme will help improve overall digestion and relieve gas and indigestion.

Possible Benefits

Improves digestion of protein as well as fats, carbohydrates, and vegetable fiber.
Reduces allergic reactions.
Enhances absorption of nutrients.

How to Use It

There are many different brands of digestive enzymes, and there may be slight variations in how to take them depending on the product. In general, take two pills or tablets fifteen minutes before each meal or snack.

Caution

Do not use digestive enzymes if you have ulcers. If you have pancreatitis, use digestive enzymes only if they are prescribed by your physician.

DONG QUAI

Dong quai *(Angelica sinesis)* has been dubbed the "female ginseng" because it is a popular Chinese remedy for common female ailments ranging from menstrual cramps to PMS to hot flashes. So why I am writing about this herb in a book on allergies? Traditional Chinese healers often include dong quai in their combination herbal formulas to treat respiratory symptoms due to allergy and colds. Dong quai is an expectorant that helps loosen mucus and ease congestion. It contains compounds that relax smooth muscle tissue, which not only helps soothe menstrual cramps, but can also relieve spasms that irritate the bronchial passages and produce unproductive, dry, hacking coughs.

Possible Benefits

Relieves tightness in chest due to allergic symptoms.
Natural expectorant.

How to Use It

Look for an antiallergy formula containing dong quai.

Caution

Dong quai should not be used by pregnant women, or by menstruating women who have unusually heavy flow. Dong quai can also cause photosensitivity to the sun, which means you should limit your exposure to the sun while you are taking this herb.

VITAMIN E

Vitamin E is a fat-soluble antioxidant that through the years has been touted as a cure-all for virtually all ills, from infertility to heart disease to cancer. I'm not promising that vitamin E will cure your allergy and asthma, but it should help relieve your symptoms. More important, if you aren't getting enough of this vitamin, it may even worsen your symptoms and increase susceptibility to developing allergies. Vitamin E reduces levels of IgE, the antibody that is produced by the body when it is exposed to an allergen. Elevated levels of IgE are also associated with asthma. Therefore, reducing IgE may help to both relieve allergic symptoms and lower the risk of having an asthma attack. Vitamin E is also an antihistamine and a potent anti-inflammatory. It inhibits the biological pathway in the body that triggers inflammation and is responsible for the damage to the lungs inflicted by asthma. Low levels of vitamin E are linked to a worsening of wheezing in asthmatic patients.

Take note moms-to-be. In one intriguing study conducted at Aberdeen University, in Scotland, researchers found that children whose mothers had the highest intake of vitamin E in their diet during pregnancy were less sensitive to common allergens (such as pollen and dust mites) than those born to mothers with a low intake of vitamin E. Good food sources of vitamin E include nuts, leafy green vegetables, and vegetable oils.

Possible Benefits

Protects against free radical damage.
Reduces allergic symptoms.
Protects against asthma.
Prevents inflammation.

How to Use It

Take one (400 mg) capsule of dry succinate E-complex (alpha and gamma tocopherol plus tocotrienols) up to twice daily, or take a multivitamin containing this E-complex.

ELDERBERRY

Elderberry *(Sambucus nigra)* is a time-honored remedy to treat colds, flus, and respiratory infections. A much-publicized Israeli study showed that people infected with the influenza virus who took elderberry recovered significantly faster than those who did not, and had less severe symptoms. Test tube studies of elderberry have shown that it has strong antiviral properties: It kills viruses by preventing them from penetrating the cells of the body. Since viruses cannot reproduce unless they have attached themselves to another cell, they quickly die off. Although there have not been any studies on elderberry and allergy, this herb is included in many combination antiallergy formulas. Based on the study of flu patients, we know that elderberry can reduce respiratory symptoms due to a viral infection; it's reasonable to assume that it may have a similar effect when those symptoms are due to allergy. Elderberry is rich in flavonoids, which in addition to being potent antioxidants, may help stabilize immune function and inhibit the release of histamine by mast cells. Elderberry is also a natural anti-inflammatory, which can help soothe irritated nasal passages.

Possible Benefits

Relieves allergic symptoms.
Thins out mucus.
Antiviral.

How to Use It

Take one (500 mg) capsule twice daily, or look for an antiallergy combination formula containing elderberry. For dry, scratchy irritated throats, take one teaspoonful of elderberry syrup.

ELECAMPANE

Known by the botanical name of *Inula helenium*, this herb has been used for centuries by healers worldwide as a treatment for common respiratory ailments, including asthma and bronchitis. Although there are no clinical studies confirming its effectiveness for these conditions, when a supplement has been used consistently for one purpose for a significant period of time, it's reasonable to assume that there's something to it. Today, it is included in many combination antiallergy herbal formulas. It contains two compounds, inulin and mucilage, which provide a soothing coating along the respiratory tract. In Europe, elecampane is treated as strong medicine, and is not available without a prescription. Although it is sold over the counter here, I recommend that before using it (or any herbal preparation, for the matter) you work with a knowledgeable health-care provider, especially if you are under treatment for asthma. This herb is also used to treat indigestion and intestinal parasites.

Possible Benefits

Relieves coughs from bronchitis and asthma.

How to Use It

Take one-half to one teaspoon (3 ml) of tincture (extract) up to three times daily, or drink a cup of elecampane tea up to three times daily.

EPHEDRA

Ephedra *(Ephedra sinica)* is best known today as the key ingredient in several popular diet pills. It is often combined with aspirin and caffeine to rev up metabolism and burn fat (the so-called aspirin "stack" that you read about in diet and bodybuilding magazines). Despite its widespread use, ephedra is one of the most controversial herbs on the market today. There have been numerous health warnings about taking high doses of ephedra because it can raise blood pressure and place an unhealthy burden on the heart. What is even more distressing is that teenagers have been abusing ephedra to get high. What you may not know is that ephedra has been used for thousands of years in traditional Chinese medicine as a treatment for allergy, asthma, colds, and other respiratory infections.

In fact, ephedrine and pseudoephedrine, two common ingredients in allergy and cold medicines, are synthetic versions of ephedra, and are both decongestants and bronchodilators. Ephedra is also known as Mormon tea because pioneers in the West used it as a treatment for colds.

Ephedra is found in many herbal combination formulas for colds, flus, and allergy, and I'm frequently asked whether it is safe. My answer is, it depends on what you're using it for, and how you're using it, and your personal medical history. First, I don't recommend ephedra for weight loss. I've seen too many people get "jumpy" and irritable on it, and I don't think it was ever intended to be used this way. However, I believe that ephedra can be an appropriate natural treatment for colds and allergies, if used correctly, that is, *under the supervision of a natural healer or physician.* There have been numerous studies confirming ephedra as an effective treatment for colds and mild asthma, and I think its long-term use as a treatment for these problems confirms that there's something to it. Studies have also confirmed that ephedra is an anti-inflammatory, which is another way of saying it helps soothe bronchial spasms and opens up constricted breathing passages.

Even in low doses, however, ephedra is not safe for people with heart conditions, people who are overly sensitive to stimulants (such as caffeine), or people with thyroid problems. Ephedra is actually a weaker version of adrenaline, the flight-or-fight hormone that supercharges the body for action. So if you have trouble sleeping, or have a nervous disposition, this herb is not for you. It's definitely not safe for people who take higher-than-recommended doses, whether they are trying to lose weight or get high. And I don't think that this herb was ever intended to be taken daily—it should only be used occasionally. If you choose to use ephedra, stick to the correct dose and stop taking it when your symptoms have improved. By the way, these same rules apply to over-the-counter cold medications with ephedralike ingredients—if you shouldn't use ephedra, you should steer clear of these products as well.

Possible Benefits

Clears congestion.
Opens up bronchial tubes.
Relieves asthma.

How to Use It

First, check with your physician to make sure that you do not have an underlying medical condition that disqualifies you from taking this herb. Drink one cup of tea to relieve cold and allergy symptoms. If you take ephedra capsules, do not exceed 24 mg of ephedrine daily.

ESSENTIAL FATTY ACIDS

It's not just your car that may need an oil change. If you suffer from asthma or allergies, you may need an oil change too! By "oil" I mean the fats you use to cook your food and dress your salads, and those in the foods that you eat. The modern diet is sorely lacking in "good fats," the essential fatty acids, which we must obtain through food because they cannot be produced by the body. There are two kinds of essential fatty acids—omega 3 fatty acids and omega 6 fatty acids. Omega 3 fatty acids are found in cold-water fatty fish (such as salmon, tuna, and mackerel) and some seeds, such as flaxseed, and grains. Omega 6 fatty acids are found in vegetable oils and nuts. We tend to get more than enough omega 6, but not enough omega 3.

Take note: Essential fatty acids are not found in red meat, pizza, french fries, snack foods, and the other dietary staples that compose the standard American diet. If you follow the typical modern diet, you are consuming huge quantities of so-called bad fat—saturated fat and transfatty acids (also called hydrogenated fats)—but not nearly enough good fat. And here's why not eating enough good fat can hurt you. Essential fatty acids are essential for a healthy immune system. These fats increase natural killer cell activity, which improve your body's ability to resist infections and cancer, but decrease prostaglandins, the hormonelike substances that trigger inflammation and can aggravate allergy and asthma symptoms. On the other hand, saturated fats and transfatty acids (produced when vegetable oils are hardened into margarine or heated for cooking) can promote inflammation. Many researchers believe that the increase in the incidence of asthma and allergy is due to the lack of good fat—and the overabundance of bad fat—in the modern diet.

So, how do you get more good fat into your life? First, clean up your diet. Eat more fatty fish (if you are not allergic to fish!) and sprinkle ground flaxseed on your cereal or yogurt. Flaxseed is sold at most natural food stores. Don't eat at fast-food restaurants (a major source of bad transfatty acids) and avoid all processed foods (such as snack foods, chips, and packaged cookies). But to really make sure that you're getting enough good fats, I recommend that you take an essential fatty acid supplement.

Essential fatty acids also protect against heart disease

and may reduce the risk of developing certain forms of cancer.

Possible Benefits

Relieves inflammation.
Normalizes immune function.
Reduces symptoms of asthma and allergy.

How to Use It

Take one capsule of essential fatty acids up to twice daily.

Sprinkle one to three tablespoons of ground flaxseed on your food daily.

EUCALYPTUS

Got a stuffy nose? Try taking a whiff of eucalyptus oil, derived from the leaf of the eucalyptus tree *(Eucalyptus globulus)*, which is native to Australia. This early form of aromatherapy has been used for thousands of years to treat nasal congestion and coughs due to allergy, colds, and flu. Eucalyptus is also an antiseptic, and can be used as a gargle for sore throats.

If you suffer from sinusitis, inflammation of the sinus membranes most often due to allergy or colds, please try the "steam therapy" described below for a day or two before loading yourself up with decongestants. It helps clear out your airways and relieves congestion without drying out your sinuses, as decongestants often do. And please, avoid asking your doctor for an antibiotic. Most cases of sinusitis are not helped by antibiotics, and can be made worse by setting the stage for a rebound infection once you stop taking the drug. Save antibiotics for when you really need them!

Possible Benefits

Clears out chest and sinuses.

How to Use It

Put one to five drops of extract in a vaporizer.

Put one to five drops of extract in a large pot of hot water. Inhale the steam from the water. Use a towel to make a tent over your head to keep the steam contained. Breathe in the steam for about ten minutes. Repeat every few hours, as needed. Be careful not to burn yourself! An old-fashioned but highly effective remedy.

Caution

Strong odors may trigger asthma attacks in susceptible people. If you find that your asthma is made worse by odors, I would not advise any form of aromatherapy.

EYEBRIGHT

Eyebright (*Euphrasia officinalis*) is a time-honored remedy for burning, itchy, irritated eyes due to cold or allergy. Eyebright, a natural anti-inflammatory, is rich in flavonoids, chemicals that can help block the release of histamine by mast cells, which is what causes the annoying symptoms associated with an allergic reaction. Taken internally, eyebright may relieve nasal congestion, but this herb is primarily used as an eyewash. Use only prepackaged eyedrop products containing eyebright made by reputable manufacturers. Don't try making your own! You don't want to risk putting anything in your eye that could trigger a bacterial infection. In my experience, eyebright eyedrops are wonderful for soothing irritated, sore eyes due to allergy or pollution.

Possible Benefits

Relieves allergic eyes.

How to Use It

Look for a combination antiallergy formula containing eyebright.

If you need to use an eyewash, please use a sterile, prepackaged extract or combination product purchased at a reputable natural food store. Follow the directions on the label. In most cases, you will be instructed to put a specified amount of eyebright in an eye cup and wash out your eye three or four times daily. Be very careful to keep the eye cup and eyebright product clean and wash your hands carefully before touching your eyes. If you have a discharge from your eye, or if your eyes are very sore, itchy, and red, call your doctor before using any eye product.

FENUGREEK

Fenugreek *(Trigonella foenumgraecum),* a longtime remedy for colds and sore throats, is now being rediscovered as a treatment for seasonal allergies. It's usually found in antiallergy combination formulas, but may be used alone on occasion to treat particular health problems. For example, a cup of warm fenugreek tea is great for a sore throat. It contains mucilage, a spongy material that when combined with water swells into a gel, thereby providing a smooth coating for an irritated, dry throat. Rich in flavonoids, fenugreek can also thin out mucus and soothe inflamed mucous membranes.

Fenugreek has anti-inflammatory action, which also helps relieve allergy symptoms and sinus headaches. Some herbal healers use fenugreek for arthritis, another condition aggravated by inflammation. This herb contains steroidlike compounds that relieve pain; in fact, in the nineteenth century, Lydia E. Pinkham's famous Vegetable Compound for women's complaints contained a hefty dose of fenugreek. It can also reduce blood sugar levels and, therefore, may help to prevent diabetes.

Possible Benefits

Relieves scratchy throat.
Good for sinus problems.
Natural anti-inflammatory.

How to Use It

Drink one cup of fenugreek tea daily.

Look for an antiallergy combination formula containing fenugreek.

Caution

Pregnant women should not use fenugreek.

FEVERFEW

Feverfew *(Chrysanthemum parthenium),* a member of the sunflower family, is best known as a treatment for migraine headaches and has been used in natural medicine since ancient Roman times. Migraines are triggered by the release of two inflammatory substances in the body—serotonin from platelets and prostaglandins from white blood cells, which constrict blood vessels. These same substances may set off an autoimmune response that not only causes these painful headaches, but can lead to an allergic reaction. Studies of extracts from feverfew show that it inhibits the production of these and other potentially irritating chemicals, thereby preventing inflammation from spreading.

Feverfew is a common ingredient in antiallergy combination formulas. It may not relieve conventional allergy symptoms as well as other front-line supplements, but I think it can be of great benefit to people who find that their migraine headaches worsen during allergy season.

As you may have guessed from its name, feverfew can also reduce a fever.

Possible Benefits

Natural anti-inflammatory.
Relieves migraine headaches.

How to Use It

Look for an antiallergy combination formula containing feverfew.

Caution

Feverfew can interfere with blood clotting and should not be used with anticoagulant medication without first checking with your physician. Do not use during pregnancy.

FLAVONOIDS

Flavonoids are a group of more than four thousand different compounds found in plant pigments—they are the chemicals that gives plants, flowers, fruits, and vegetables their vibrant colors. Only fifty or so are found in commonly consumed foods, such as oranges, apples, lemon, soy foods, onions, berries, red grapes, and tea. About half of all flavonoids are antioxidants, but they're important for other reasons. Flavonoids slow the breakdown of vitamin C in the body, which prevents vitamin C from being used up too quickly. In fact, if you take vitamin C supplements, you will notice that many brands include flavonoids to help enhance their effectiveness. Since vitamin C is also important for boosting glutathione, another important antioxidant in the body, at least indirectly, flavonoids are responsible for maintaining healthy levels of both vitamin C and glutathione.

Some of the most popular herbs, such as ginkgo and grape seed extract, owe their healing properties to their flavonoid content.

For allergy sufferers, flavonoids can be a godsend. First, they strengthen small blood vessels called capillaries, which help protect cells from foreign particles (such as allergens) by forming a protective barrier. Second, flavonoids reduce inflammation typical of allergies and help normalize immune function, which reduces allergy symptoms. In particular, flavonoids help stabilize mast cells, the immune cells that produce histamine when they encounter an allergen. Flavonoids calm down these overly excited cells, preventing the release of histamine, which is responsible for those annoying allergy symptoms. Last but not least, by maintaining optimal antioxidant levels in the body, flavonoids help the body cleanse itself of pollution, toxins, and other chemicals that can send the immune system into overdrive and trigger an allergic reaction.

Flavonoids are not just good for allergies, they help protect against both cancer and heart disease. Numerous studies have documented that people who eat a diet rich in flavonoids (primarily fruits and vegetables) have a significantly reduced risk of heart disease and many different forms of cancer than those who do not.

There are several different forms of flavonoids on the market. Combination flavonoids are sold separately, with vitamin C, or in antiallergy products. Some flavonoids are so effective against allergy (quercetin and proanthocyanins

[PCOs]) that they are sold individually. These tend to be pricier than the generic bioflavonoid products, but are often more effective.

Possible Benefits

Relieves allergic symptoms.
Improves blood circulation.
Reduces inflammation.
Normalizes immune cells.

How to Use It

Take one (2,500 mg) capsule of mixed citrus flavonoids daily.

FORSKOLIN

Forskolin is an extract of the herb *Coleus forskohili,* long used in Ayurvedic medicine to treat asthma and allergies. It is a natural muscle relaxant, which can help soothe bronchial spasms typical of asthma and bronchitis. In at least two studies, inhaled forskolin was shown to be as effective as bronchodilator drugs found in prescription inhalers. Taken orally, it would have the same effect, only slower.

Forskolin has also been used to treat high blood pressure and glaucoma (high blood pressure in the eye). Recently, it has also been studied as a potential anticancer drug.

Forskolin is sold separately and included in combination formulas for allergy. This herb can boost levels of thyroid hormone, which is good if you are hypothyroid or low in thyroid hormone, but can be bad if you are hyperthyroid or have too much thyroid hormones. Forskolin can also cause a sudden drop in blood pressure, and is not good for people with low or erratic blood pressure. Forskolin is strong medicine, which is why it's so effective, but in my opinion, it should only be used under the direction of a nutritionally oriented physician. If you are taking other medication, please check with your physician before using a product containing forskolin.

Possible Benefits

Relieves symptoms of asthma.

How to Use It

Work with a knowledgeable nutritionally oriented physician or natural healer to determine the right dose for you.

GARLIC

A chopped-up garlic clove mixed with a bit of honey is an old-time remedy for bronchitis, sore throats, and other respiratory infections. Garlic (*Allium sativum*) can reduce mucus buildup in the airways and lungs and relieve congestion. Today, garlic extract or specific components from garlic are often added to antiallergy combination formulas. Garlic contains powerful sulphur compounds (the chemicals that give it its telltale pungent odor) that are a virtual natural pharmacy. It is also rich in quercetin, a flavonoid well-known for its antiallergy properties (see page 97). Garlic is a potent anti-inflammatory; it slows down the production of prostaglandins and leukotrienes, which promote inflammation in the body and can worsen asthma symptoms. Garlic is also antibacterial and antifungal. It is one of the few natural substances that is effective against candida albicans, the fungus that causes yeast infections. Where's the allergy link? Many natural healers believe that in some people, chronic yeast infections may overexcite the immune system, leaving it vulnerable to autoimmune problems such as allergy. Garlic is also an excellent source of selenium, an important antioxidant that may help protect against asthma (see page 101). In addition, garlic is good for your heart and may help the liver detoxify chemicals that can cause cancer. Cooked garlic is an excellent blood thinner. For all of these reasons, I recommend that people eat garlic or take garlic supplements.

Possible Benefits

Natural anti-inflammatory.
Microbe fighter—antibacterial, antiviral, antiyeast.
Reduces mucus buildup.

How to Use It

Take one (500 mg) aged, odorless garlic capsule daily.

Caution

As good as garlic is, some people are allergic to it. If you are, avoid products that contain garlic.

GINGER ROOT

Used in the traditional Chinese medicine (TCM) system for thousands of years, ginger *(Zingiber officinale)* is becoming a popular antiallergy treatment in the West. Ginger, best known as an anti-inflammatory, has been well studied in laboratories throughout the world. In recent years, scientists have learned that ginger inhibits the production of leukotrienes, the immune cells that trigger inflammation. It also contains two oils, gingerols and shogaols, which relax smooth muscle tissue. As many of you know, ginger is often used to treat nausea and stomach cramps, but the same type of smooth muscle tissue that lines the gastrointestinal tract also lines the respiratory tract, and, similarly, can go into spasm if irritated by allergens or other toxins. Ginger relieves tightness in the chest typical of asthma, bronchitis, and other respiratory problems by dilating (relaxing) the bronchial tubes.

Many common allergy remedies today can leave you feeling tired, dizzy, or lightheaded. The problem is, many allergy sufferers feel "spaced out" to begin with, especially during bad pollen days. In contrast, ginger is also an excellent treatment for dizziness or motion sickness. I take a ginger capsule every day to prevent arthritis, a condition that is also aggravated by inflammation.

Ginger comes in many different shapes and forms,

from fresh grated ginger, to ginger tea, to dried ginger capsules, to combination antiallergy products that include ginger. And as sushi fans know, grated ginger is often served along with sushi. Notice I did not mention ginger ale: The popular soft drink does not contain enough ginger to be effective, and has way too much sugar.

Possible Benefits

Relieves inflammation that aggravates allergy symptoms.

Soothes bronchial tubes.

How to Use It

Look for a combination antiallergy formula containing powdered ginger root extract.

Have a cup of ginger tea (packaged tea bags are sold in natural food stores and some supermarkets).

Eat a slice of fresh ginger.

Caution

Ginger can be a blood thinner, which helps prevent strokes. However, if you are taking other medication or having surgery, be sure to tell your doctor that you are taking a ginger supplement. You will need to discontinue taking the supplement before the surgery.

GINKGO

Ginkgo *(Ginkgo biloba)* is the oldest living species of tree, with some trees living more than one thousand years. Although it is best known as the herb for the brain, for thousands of years traditional Chinese healers have used the leaf and fruit of the ginkgo tree to treat coughs, asthma, and inflammatory conditions, including allergy. Knowledgeable natural healers still prescribe ginkgo for these same problems today. Of course, unlike healers of the past who relied on intuition and trial and error, we now have a better understanding of how ginkgo works. In fact, it is one of the most carefully studied of all the herbs.

Ginkgo is a powerful antioxidant that can defeat some of the strongest free radicals on the planet, including superoxide and the hydroxy radical, both of which are capable of inflicting great damage on the cells and tissues of the body. It is also an anti-inflammatory—special chemicals in ginkgo called ginkgolides inhibit PAF (platelet activating factor), which is involved in both triggering the body's allergy response and the resulting inflammation. In a study of asthmatic patients published in *Prostaglandins,* a medical journal, a ginkgo biloba extract dramatically reduced bronchial restriction for up to six hours in patients who had been exposed to an allergen that normally triggered an asthmatic response.

Ginkgo improves microcirculation, that is, it increases blood flow to small vessels, which is often impaired by asthma. It helps regulate a chemical found in the body called nitric oxide, which improves the muscular tone of blood vessels, thereby enhancing blood flow. Rich in flavonoids such as quercetin and proanthocyanins, ginkgo offers significant protection against allergic reactions.

Ginkgo offers some amazing side benefits. In addition to improving mental performance, it protects against atherosclerosis (hardening of the arteries) and is a natural blood thinner, which helps prevent strokes. And unlike standard allergy medications that may make you sleepy, ginkgo makes you more alert. Feel free to drive or operate heavy machinery after taking this amazing herb!

Possible Benefits

Blocks allergic reactions.
Prevents inflammation.
Improves circulation.

How to Use It

Take one (60 mg) capsule or tablet daily. Ginkgo is included in many antiallergy combination formulas.

Caution

Since ginkgo can be a blood thinner, be sure to tell your doctor you are taking ginkgo if you are undergoing surgery, or taking other prescription heart drugs.

GRAPE SEED EXTRACT

Grape seed extract is a rich source of antioxidant flavonoids called proanthocyanins (PCOs) also found in the blue, purple, and green pigments of plants and pine bark extract. Grape seed extract is a natural antihistamine that is believed to prevent the release of histamine by mast cells, thereby blocking potential allergic reactions to allergens. It is also a potent antioxidant and anti-inflammatory. For the past two decades, grape seed extract has been touted as an antiallergy supplement, and there is a lot of anecdotal evidence to support this claim. However, grape seed extract did not fare well in a recent study conducted at the allergy research lab at the University of Cincinnati. In this study of forty-nine hay fever patients, researchers did not find any difference in symptom relief or the need to use "rescue" medication among allergic patients taking grape seed extract (100 mg twice daily) or a placebo for two months immediately before or during allergy season. Frankly, I'm not surprised. Herbal supplements like grape seed extract are best used to prevent allergies before the fact, and should not be first used during allergy season. These supplements work by preventing the cascade of events that lead to an allergic reaction—to be fully effective, they should be taken months before allergy season begins. In my experience, the right supplements can significantly diminish allergy symptoms if taken for a long enough period. Also, I feel that these supplements are meant to work in synergy with other supplements. For example, grape seed extract, rich in flavonoids, should be taken with vitamin C, green tea extract, and other antioxidants and flavonoids to enhance its effectiveness. I would love to see a study investigating the *long-term effect* on allergies of using a combination formula containing grape seed extracts and other powerful antiallergy supplements.

Grape seed extract has many other health benefits

worth mentioning. Among other things, grape seed extract may lower cholesterol levels, prevent blood clots, lower blood pressure, and protect cells against mutations that can cause cancerous changes.

Possible Benefits

Relieves hay fever symptoms.
Reduces inflammatory response.
Protects against free radical attack.

How to Use It

Take one (100 mg) tablet twice daily. I take grape seed extract in combination with green tea extract, which is the next supplement down.

GREEN TEA

Allergy symptoms dragging you down? Try sipping a cup of green tea *(Camellia sinensis)* or taking a green tea supplement. A cup of green tea, which contains about half the caffeine of a comparable amount of coffee, will give you a mild boost. (If you're caffeine-sensitive, look for brands of green tea that are decaffeinated.) Green tea is also rich in a special type of bioflavonoid called catechins, which are natural antihistamines. In addition, green tea contains powerful antioxidants. Since green tea is more lightly processed than black tea, it contains more beneficial flavonoids, which can be destroyed during heating and other processing techniques. Green tea can be used alone or may be included in antiallergy combination supplements.

More good news about green tea. Numerous studies have shown that compounds found in green tea can inhibit the growth of cancerous tumors in animals. Population studies suggest that green tea offers protection against lung cancer, even among smokers. For example, Japanese men are heavier smokers than men in the United States, yet the rate for lung cancer in Japan is lower than in the United States. (This is not to suggest that it's safe to smoke—it's probably the worst thing you can do for your health in general, and your allergies in particular.)

Possible Benefits

May relieve allergic symptoms.
Protects against free radicals.

How to Use It

Drink a cup of green tea. If caffeine bothers you, be sure to buy the decaffeinated variety. Take one or two green tea tablets daily.

GUMWEED

Gumweed *(Grindelia camporum),* also known as grindalia, gum plant, and tar weed, is a time-honored remedy for asthma, bronchitis, whooping cough (which has been virtually eliminated in the West due to vaccination), and any respiratory condition that results in a chronic, hacking cough. It is a natural muscle relaxant that targets the smooth muscle of the respiratory tract, thereby helping to prevent spasms typical of asthma and bronchitis. It also lowers blood pressure, which is good if you have high blood pressure, but may be too sedating for people with low blood pressure. Gumweed is included in several antiallergy combination formulas, often with other traditional remedies such as elecampane and lobelia. Herbalists warn that in high doses, gumweed can cause kidney problems and stomach upset, so stick within the recommended range. Gumweed is also used in homeopathic remedies for allergy.

Possible Benefits

Relieves bronchial spasms.

How to Use It

Look for an antiallergy combination formula containing gumweed.

HISTIDINE

Histidine is an amino acid, a building block of protein. There are twenty-two different amino acids, fourteen of which can be made by the body, and eight, called essential amino acids, which must be obtained through food. Histidine is classified as an essential amino acid for infants, but not for adults. But if you suffer from allergies, histidine may be essential for you! In the body, histidine is used to manufacture histamine, the substance released by mast cells that causes the nasty symptoms associated with allergy, such as watery eyes and a stuffy nose. At first glance, it would appear as if histidine is our enemy in the allergy wars, but in fact, it is an ally. Histidine helps dampen the inflammatory response that is triggered by histamine release, thereby reducing the irritation caused by the allergen. Histidine is a common ingredient in antiallergy combination formulas, and it is often teamed with garlic, horseradish, and other herbs and supplements.

Due to its anti-inflammatory properties, histidine is also used as a natural treatment for rheumatoid arthritis, which, like allergy, is an autoimmune condition caused by an overzealous immune system that attacks the joints of the body.

Possible Benefits

Reduces inflammation.
Relieves allergic response.

How to Use It

Find a combination antiallergy formula containing 50 mg histidine.

HORSERADISH

Chopped horseradish root (*Amoracia lapathifolia*) is both a condiment and a medicinal herb widely used throughout the world. In Eastern Europe, horseradish is served with fish and stews; in Japan, a form of horseradish called wasabi is served with sushi. If you've ever eaten horseradish, you know that the instant you bite into this herb, you feel a stinging, warm sensation that seems to go right through your throat up to your sinuses. Within seconds, your nose begins to run, and you may even start coughing. No wonder for centuries healers have used horseradish to clear out clogged sinuses or a congested chest due to colds, allergies, and other respiratory problems. It is an excellent expectorant and mild antiseptic, which is probably one of the reasons why the Japanese eat wasabi with raw fish, which may contain bacteria that would be killed in the cooking process.

Extract of dried horseradish root is used in combination antiallergy formulas. Of course, those of you who are more adventurous can use the fresh root, which is sold in the refrigerated section of many supermarkets and gourmet shops.

Possible Benefits

Helps to clear nose and chest.

How to Use It

Find a combination formula containing dried horseradish root.

Mix two tablespoons of grated root with small amount of honey and warm water.

Take one tablespoon twice daily.

JEWELWEED

If you spend any time outdoors, either gardening in your backyard or hiking in the woods, this is one natural remedy that you should keep close at hand. Jewelweed *(Impatiens capensis)* is a plant that grows in the wild. The juice from the stem is a time-honored remedy for the itchy, burning rash caused by contact with poison ivy, oak, and sumac, all of which contain a chemical called urushiol, which is a potent allergen. There is no cure that will magically heal these rashes, but commercial skin lotion and soap derived from jewelweed may help take the edge off. Jewelweed is also recommended for skin abrasions due to bug bites. Jewelweed products are sold in sporting good stores and natural food stores and on the Internet.

Possible Benefits

Reduces irritation due to urushiol rash.

How to Use It

Lather up with jewelweed soap in the shower. Leave on your skin for thirty seconds, then rinse off.

Apply liquid spray directly to affected area three times daily.

Caution

Some people may be allergic to jewelweed. Don't wait to find out after your body is covered with a poison ivy rash! After purchasing the product, apply a small amount of jewelweed soap or lotion to your upper arm. Leave it on for twenty-four hours. If the area becomes red and irritated, do not use this product.

LICORICE

In the United States, licorice is best known as a sweet flavored candy, but in reality, licorice root *(Glycyrrhiza glabra)* is one of the most popular herbal medicines in the world. It's a mainstay of the traditional Chinese medicine system and for thousands of years, it's been used to treat asthma, allergy, colds, and flus, among other conditions. It's also widely used in Western Europe. Licorice is a rich source of flavonoids, which are potent antioxidants. It is also an anti-inflammatory, although not directly. It contains a chemical called glycyrrhizin that blocks an enzyme that breaks down cortisone, the body's natural anti-inflammatory, thereby enhancing its effectiveness. Cortisone is similar to steroid medications that are prescribed for severe asthma and allergy. Licorice is a common ingredient in cough syrup: It coats the throat in a protective covering that both soothes irritation and promotes healing. It is also an excellent expectorant, which can help clear a congested chest. The great seventeenth-century herbalist Culpeper wrote that licorice "was a fine medicine for hoarseness." To add to its accomplishments, licorice has strong antiviral properties and is being seriously studied by scientists as a potential therapy against cancer. It is also used to treat symptoms of menopause.

However, there's a downside to glycyrrhizin—it increases the level of another hormone in the body that can also raise blood pressure. Therefore, people with untreated high blood pressure or heart disease should avoid licorice. (There is a special form of licorice, deglycyrrhizinated licorice root, or DGL, that does not contain glycyrrhizin and is used as a treatment for ulcers, but it is not effective against allergy.)

Licorice should only be used short-term to treat acute symptoms. People who take licorice can retain salt and lose potassium (which is one way that licorice causes high blood pressure), so if you take a supplement with licorice, be sure to eat lots of fresh fruits and vegetables to replenish lost potassium. If you use licorice, I prefer that you do so under the supervision of a knowledgeable physician or natural healer. Licorice is strong medicine, and it can be good medicine if used correctly.

Possible Benefits

Anti-inflammatory.
Great for coughs due to colds or allergy.

How to Use It

Take three (250 mg) capsules of dried powder daily, or a daily dose equivalent to a total of 200 to 400 mg of glycyrrhizin.

Caution

Pregnant women or women with PMS, particularly those who retain fluid, and people with kidney disease, heart disease, or untreated high blood pressure should not use licorice. Do not take this herb for more than two weeks unless directed by your physician.

LOBELIA

Lobelia *(Lobelia inflata)* is also known as pukeweed (in very high doses, it induces vomiting) and Indian tobacco. This herb has been touted as a cure for tobacco addiction, although this claim has never been proven. Used by herbal healers in Europe and the United States for hundreds of years—it was a popular herb among Native Americans— lobelia is a standard traditional remedy for asthma and bronchitis. It is both a muscle relaxant and an expectorant, which works particularly well for conditions such as bronchitis that can be aggravated by mucus buildup in the chest and airways. Today, lobelia is most often combined with other herbs, such as gumweed and cayenne, in antiallergy combination formulas. Lobeline is the active ingredient. Natural healers use lobeline to treat nicotine addiction; it is reputed to reduce the urge to smoke.

Possible Benefits

Good expectorant.

How to Use It

Stick to combination antiallergy formulas containing lobelia.

Caution

Do not use lobelia if you are pregnant or breast feeding. In very high doses, this herb can cause nausea and vomiting and can be toxic. Your best bet is to stick to antiallergy combination formulas.

LUNGWORT

Lungwort *(Pulmonaria officinalis)* is hardly a household name these days, but I bet your great-grandmother knew all about it. And so do modern-day herbalists, who are using it as part of the herbal armamentarium to defeat allergy symptoms. As you can tell from its name, lungwort is a time-honored remedy for bronchitis, upper respiratory infections, and bad coughs. It contains flavonoids such as quercetin, and other anti-inflammatory chemicals that relieve allergy symptoms. It is also an expectorant, which helps to clear the lungs. You may find lungwort tea or dried powder at a well-stocked natural food store. It is most often used in antiallergy herbal formulas in combination with other time-honored healing herbs such as mullein.

Possible Benefits

Relieves upper respiratory infections.
Natural anti-inflammatory.

How to Use It

Make yourself a cup of lungwort tea. Steep one table-spoon of dried, powdered herb in hot water. Strain. Drink one cup daily. Or look for an antiallergy combination formula containing lungwort.

MAGNESIUM

Magnesium is a mineral that is critical for a healthy body. It's involved in scores of vital tasks ranging from the production of ATP, the fuel that runs the cells, to the formation of bone, to the production of key proteins, to the beating of the heart. Magnesium is found in whole grains, nuts, seeds, and vegetables. The problem is, the Western diet is notoriously low in magnesium. In particular, processed foods, which are the mainstay of the modern diet, are stripped of such nutrients as magnesium, resulting in a less than optimal magnesium intake. Excess consumption of caffeine, soda, alcohol, and sugar can further deplete your magnesium stores. Many nutritionally oriented physicians believe that low levels of magnesium may leave us more vulnerable to developing asthma and allergies. In fact, asthmatics typically have low magnesium levels.

Natural healers routinely prescribe magnesium supplements to treat asthma and allergic conditions. Magnesium, which is involved in the contraction of smooth muscle tissue, can help relax irritated bronchial tubes, relieving spasms and opening the airways.

In addition, magnesium is a mild antihistamine and

can reduce allergy symptoms, which, in some cases, can trigger asthma attacks.

Magnesium is also used to treat numerous common ailments including high blood pressure, angina, stress-related disorders, heart disease, and chronic fatigue syndrome.

Possible Benefits

Relieves tightness in chest due to bronchial spasms.
May dampen allergic response.
Good for stress.

How to Use It

Magnesium works best when combined with another essential mineral, calcium. Take one capsule or pill containing 250 mg of magnesium in the form of glycinated magnesite and 500 mg of calcium twice or three times daily. I call this combination "nature's tranquilizer." But don't worry, it won't make you drowsy!

Caution

Some people may find that magnesium causes diarrhea. If your stomach gets upset, cut back on your dose.

MARSHMALLOW

Sorry, I'm not talking about the soft, white gooey candy so popular today. I'm talking about the marshmallow plant

(Althea officinalis), which has been used to treat coughs and colds for more than a thousand years. Marshmallow is rich in mucilage, a substance that, when combined with water, forms a gel that soothes and protects the throat. It is also a good expectorant. Marshmallow is also a time-honored remedy for gastrointestinal woes such as ulcers and colitis. If you suffer from both allergy and GI distress, this herb may be the herb for you! Marshmallow is included in herbal antiallergy combination formulas.

Possible Benefits

Good for sore, dry throat.
Helps relieve cough.
Good for ulcers.

How to Use It

Drink a cup of marshmallow tea daily. Look for an antiallergy combination containing marshmallow.

MILK THISTLE

The milk thistle plant *(Silybum marianum)*—primarily its seeds—is best known as the herb for liver health, but is also a traditional remedy for psoriasis, a skin rash that may be triggered, if not aggravated, by allergies. The active ingredient in milk thistle is silymarin, a potent antioxidant and anti-inflammatory. Conventional physicians would dismiss the connection between liver and allergy, but the fact is, it makes a lot of sense. The liver is where toxins are detoxified by the body. If the liver is not functioning at its peak, or is damaged (as in the case of cirrhosis of the liver or hepatitis), higher-than-normal levels of toxins are allowed to accumulate in the body. Excess toxins can send the immune system into overdrive, disrupting normal immune function, and can also contribute to inflammation, especially in the GI system. Studies have shown that people with both eczema and psoriasis have higher-than-normal levels of endotoxins in their bloodstream, a sign that their liver function is not up to par. Here's the allergy connection—allergy by definition is an immune system out of control. Allergy is also aggravated by inflammation. Any herb that can both reduce toxins and relieve inflammation is going to have a positive effect on the immune system, thereby reducing the risk of an allergic reaction. Many well-known natural healers advocate the use of milk thistle for people with allergy-related skin conditions, especially psoriasis, and have had good clinical experience using it. Milk thistle can also raise levels of glutathione, an important antioxidant that protects the body from free radical attack and inflammation.

In recent years, milk thistle has been touted as a treatment for serious liver disease, including liver cancer. If you have a liver problem, you should be under the care of a physician, ideally one who will incorporate helpful natural therapies with conventional medicine. But please, don't try to treat a serious medical condition on your own.

If you have been exposed to high levels of toxins, that is, you live or work in a polluted area, milk thistle may help your body better handle the toxic load.

Possible Benefits

Reduces inflammation.
Enhances liver health.
Traditional treatment for psoriasis and eczema.

How to Use It

The dose of milk thistle is based on its silymarin content. Take one capsule (140 mg silymarin) twice daily. Use a standardized extract. Please note that the dose of milk thistle is higher for liver disease. Check with your physician or natural healer.

MSM (METHYL SULFONYL METHANE)

MSM is a form of organic sulphur found in nature that plays a key role in the human body. It is essential for the production of amino acids, the building blocks of protein, and is needed to make connective tissue (such as cartilage and collagen), enzymes, antibodies, and glutathione, the body's main antioxidant. MSM is found in meat, eggs, poultry, and dairy products but because it is rapidly used up by the body, we may not get enough of it through diet alone. MSM supplements are available to fill the gap. In recent years, MSM has been touted as a treatment for a wide range of ailments from allergy to arthritis to gut problems to hair loss. In my experience, it is one of the most effective supplements on the market, especially when it comes to allergy. Studies conducted at the University of Oregon have shown that MSM may significantly reduce allergy symptoms and the need for medication in severely allergic people who are exposed to environmental allergens, such as dust mites, pollen, and animal hair. In some cases, it even reduced the symptoms associated with allergies to common foods, such as milk, shrimp, and citrus fruits. I'm not recommending that you throw caution to the wind and assume you can eat whatever you like if you take MSM. Not at all! When it comes to a food allergy, avoidance is still the best medicine, but even under the best circumstances, you may end up inadvertently eating a food that you are allergic to, and it's nice to know that MSM may reduce your allergic response. I personally have recommended MSM along with vitamin C and other flavonoids to allergic friends and family members during hay fever season, and have found that in virtually every case, within a few weeks, symptoms such as watery eyes and runny nose were eliminated. Researchers believe that MSM coats the mucous membranes of the body, forming a physical barrier against allergens and pollutants that could trigger an allergic reaction. In addition, MSM is a natural anti-inflammatory.

MSM is a nontoxic, nonallergic substance. Let me clear up one point of possible confusion. MSM is a sulphur compound. It is not related to sulfa drugs. If you are allergic to sulfa drugs, it doesn't mean that you are allergic to MSM. MSM is not plant based, which makes it a good treatment choice for allergy sufferers who are particularly sensitive to plant pollen and should avoid herbal supplements.

As noted earlier, allergy sufferers frequently have gastrointestinal problems. If you find that you are constantly popping antacids to quell excess stomach acid, MSM can help control hyperacidity at the same time it is helping to keep your allergy symptoms at bay.

Possible Benefits

Reduces symptoms of indoor and outdoor allergies.
Relieves inflammation in mucous membranes.
May help the body better cope with food allergies.
Good nonbotanical alternative to herbs.

How to Use It

MSM comes in tablets or powder. Take 1000 mg of MSM along with 500 mg of vitamin C plus flavonoids three times daily.

Mix one-quarter to three-quarters teaspoon of powder in eight ounces of water or juice. Drink three glasses daily with meals.

MULLEIN

Mullein *(Verbascum thapsus)* is a long-standing remedy for respiratory problems with coughs, such as bronchitis, chest colds, hay fever, and asthma. It contains anti-inflammatory flavonoids and soothing mucilage, which coats the throat and bronchial tubes, thereby relieving the irritation caused by constant coughing. It is also an expectorant, which helps create a more productive cough—you cough only when you really need to in order to clear your airways. Only the most ardent herbalists know how to use mullein these days, but fortunately, it's included in many antiallergy herbal formulas.

Possible Benefits

Relieves irritated throat.

How to Use It

Look for an antiallergy combination formula containing mullein. Well-stocked natural food stores may have dried mullein, which can be made into a tea. Steep one ounce of the dried root in one cup of hot water. Strain. Drink one cup daily.

NAC (N-ACETYL CYSTEINE)

NAC is one of the few Hot 55 Antiallergy Supplements that is powerful enough to use alone, but is also included in many combination formulas. First and foremost, NAC is a potent antioxidant. It boosts levels of glutathione, the primary antioxidant in the lower respiratory system that protects delicate lung tissue from free radicals formed by the body, and other toxins and irritants breathed in through the nose. Second, NAC is a mucolytic agent, that is, it thins out excess mucus by breaking up the sulphur bonds that hold it together. So if you're suffering from a chronically stuffy, runny nose during allergy season, or congestion in your chest, this supplement can help clear those clogged airways. NAC is so effective that an inhalant containing NAC is used to treat cystic fibrosis, a disease characterized by the formation of unusually thick mucus that can seriously threaten respiratory function. You will also find that NAC is stocked in most emergency rooms. NAC is a medically accepted treatment for acetaminophen (Tylenol) poisoning. In high doses, acetaminophen poisons the liver by depleting it of glutathione, which can be fatal. NAC helps restore the lost glutathione, thereby saving the liver, and ultimately saving lives.

Recently, Italian researchers have shown that NAC dramatically reduced the symptoms and severity of the flu in older patients who had not been vaccinated against the flu. It was particularly helpful in relieving respiratory symptoms.

Possible Benefits

Helps eliminate excess mucus.
Protects against free radical attack.
Reduces inflammation.

How to Use It

For severe congestion take three (500 mg) capsules daily. For mild symptoms, take two (500 mg) capsules daily, or look for a combination antiallergy formula containing NAC.

PERILLA OIL

Although it is new to the West, Asian herbalists have long used perilla leaf *(Perilla frutescens)* to treat respiratory ailments, such as coughs, colds, flus, and asthma. According to Chinese healers, perilla has a warm, soothing effect on the lungs. They recommend it to control excess mucus production, nasty coughs, and troublesome allergy symptoms. Compared to other plant-based oils, perilla oil is extremely rich in omega 3 fatty acids, the good essential fats that help reduce inflammation and quiet an overactive immune system. In contrast, the modern Western diet is abundant in omega 6 fatty acids, found in corn, soy, and other vegetable oils, that can promote inflammation. To add to its many benefits, perilla also contains antioxidant flavonoids.

As with so many other time-honored remedies, researchers are now discovering that perilla holds up to scientific scrutiny. In a Japanese study published in the *International Archives of Medicine,* daily supplementation with perilla seed oil inhibited the production of leukotrienes, messenger proteins that trigger inflammation and are associated with both asthma and allergic reactions. In the study, fourteen asthmatics were given either perilla seed oil or corn oil (high in omega 6 fatty acids) daily for four weeks. Those taking the perilla oil experienced a significant reduction in leukotrienes, while those taking the corn oil showed an increase in allergic markers such as leukotrienes and allergic immunoglobulins. In addition, the perilla seed oil group had a dramatic improvement in lung function within two to four weeks. Other studies confirm that perilla oil can help relieve allergic dermatitis, nonspecific skin rashes caused by exposure to allergens. Perilla is also an antihistamine and reduces the production of immunoglobulins that can trigger an allergic response. In addition, perilla leaf and oil may help reduce allergic sensitivity to food. Interestingly, Chinese cooks frequently add perilla leaf to cook shellfish—could it be that this leaf was used to prevent allergic reactions to a food that is a common allergen?

Possible Benefits

Relieves inflammation.
Normalizes immune system.
May reduce susceptibility to food allergies.

How to Use It

Take three (200 mg) capsules daily, or take one teaspoon of oil daily.

PROBIOTICS

Probiotics, which literally mean "for life," are bacteria that live in the small and large intestines. Unlike so-called "bad" bacteria that spread disease, probiotics are "good" bacteria that aid in digestion and help to maintain health. There are over four hundred microorganisms in the intestines, including the beneficial Lactobacillus acidophilus, which is used to culture yogurt, B. Bifidum, and the yeast Saccharomyces boulardii. Good bacteria perform several vital jobs, including keeping bad bacteria under control and strengthening immune function. Some strains of good bacteria have been shown to inhibit the growth of cancerous tumors. Recent studies suggest that good bacteria may also protect against allergy and asthma.

In one study conducted in Finland, forty-six expectant mothers with a history of asthma, hay fever, or eczema were given either a placebo or a probiotic supplement (Lactobacillus GG) two to four weeks before their expected delivery dates. After the babies were born, either the mothers continued taking the supplements themselves and breast fed their children, or the children were given the good bacteria in diluted water until they were six months old. Researchers followed the children until their second birthday. They found that children exposed to the good bacteria either directly or through breast milk were 50 percent less likely to develop these allergic ailments than the children given the placebo. Why would probiotics help prevent allergy? Researchers speculate that the good bacteria somehow train the immune system to better distinguish between harmless substances and potential troublemakers. This is in keeping with the "too clean for our own good" theory of why the incidence of allergy is growing exponentially in the developed world. Other studies have shown that probiotics inhibit the production of inflammatory substances such as TNF-alpha, the protein produced by the immune system that triggers an inflammatory response.

It's not just children who benefit from probiotics—adults need them too, especially to maintain normal immune function. Numerous studies have shown that people with autoimmune diseases such as rheumatoid arthritis are deficient in good bacteria, but so are many so-called healthy people. Good bacteria thrive on a high-fiber diet, which is just the opposite of the highly refined, processed Western diet. In addition, antibiotics can kill both good and bad bacteria, which is yet another reason it's not wise to take antibiotics unless absolutely necessary. And even if you don't take antibiotics directly, antibiotics are routinely fed to livestock, and residues are routinely found in meat and dairy products (unless you buy antibiotic-free products). Even excess stress can kill off good bacteria. Therefore, it's more than likely you don't have an optimal level of good bacteria, and to make up for this shortfall, I recommend that everyone take a probiotic supplement.

Possible Benefits

Normalizes immune function.
Reduces likelihood of allergic reactions.
Helps detoxify chemicals and additives in food.
Supports gut health.

How to Use It

Take 1 tablespoon of L-acidophilus daily, or two capsules daily. Some brands of probiotics must be stored in the refrigerator.

QUERCETIN

Quercetin, a superstar among flavonoids, is a front-line treatment against allergy and asthma. It is found in the skins of apples and yellow and red onions and is also sold in capsule form. A recent study published in the *American Journal of Respiratory and Critical Care Medicine* (December 2001) found that people who eat more apples are less likely to develop asthma than those who rarely eat apples.

The researchers attributed the reduction in asthma to the flavonoid content in apples, and certainly quercetin is entitled to take some, if not all, of the credit. Although quercetin is included in many antiallergy formulas containing dozens of ingredients, it works well enough that you may find that quercetin alone is enough to keep your allergy symptoms under control. (Always take quercetin with bromelain, to aid absorption, and vitamin C, which enhances the activity of flavonoids.) Quercetin stabilizes the walls of mast cells, thereby preventing the release of histamine and serotonin, the chemicals that make you miserable during allergy season. Quercetin is also an anti-inflammatory, which will help relieve symptoms and reduce swelling in airways, which can be aggravated by allergens and asthma.

An antioxidant, quercetin prevents oxidation of LDL or bad cholesterol, which can cause a heart attack.

Possible Benefits

Relieves allergic symptoms.
Reduces risk of asthma.
Anti-inflammatory.

How to Use It

Take one (400 mg) quercetin capsule with one (100 mg) bromelain capsule and 500 mg of vitamin C with meals, up to three times daily.

REISHI MUSHROOM

Reishi mushroom *(Ganoderma lucidum)* has been used for more than two thousand years in traditional Chinese medicine, where it is known as the "medicine of kings." Listed in the renowned *Shen Nong Ben Cao Jing,* China's first herbal guide, reishi is prescribed to relieve stress and normalize the immune system, or as the Chinese call it, the "Wei Chi." Unlike Western medicine, in which the primary focus is on treating symptoms, in Chinese medicine, the focus is on preserving health and maintaining the normal balance between body systems. Reishi is one of the few herbs that can both enhance the effect of disease-fighting immune cells and dampen the action of cells that cause inflammation. Several studies have confirmed that reishi is an antihistamine, which would further relieve allergic symptoms. Similar to another highly revered herb, ginseng, reishi is taken daily as a tonic to maintain health, not to rid the body of disease.

Reishi has a calming effect on the nervous system and also contains antioxidant compounds. If you find that your allergy symptoms are stressing you out, this could be the right treatment for you.

Reishi extract is sold separately and is included in many antiallergy combination formulas. The mushroom itself is not as popular for cooking as other Asian mushrooms, such as shiitake, so you're not likely to find it in the produce section. The capsules and extract are a more potent form, and are more easily absorbed by the body.

Possible Benefits

May help to prevent allergic reactions by normalizing immune function.

Relieves stress.

Sometimes used as a treatment for insomnia.

How to Use It

Take one (500 mg) capsule daily, or use a combination antiallergy formula containing reishi mushroom.

Caution

Mushrooms are fungi, and fungi are mold. If you are allergic to mushrooms or molds, I would avoid using reishi or any other mushroom-derived product.

SARSAPARILLA

If you have eczema or psoriasis, you may think that you have a skin problem, but in reality, your problem may be all in your . . . gut! Many natural healers and progressive physicians believe there is a link between gut health and skin ailments. The common denominator is allergy.

Let me explain. People with both eczema and psoriasis have higher-than-normal levels of endotoxins in their bloodstream, waste products made by the gut from native bacteria and from our own digestion and metabolism. Endotoxins should stay in the gut, but the presence of elevated levels of endotoxins outside the gut suggests that the digestive system is not doing an adequate job in breaking down food and disposing of toxins. When endotoxins hit the bloodstream, it alerts the immune system that something is wrong. As a result, the immune system is constantly on edge, leading it to attack otherwise benign substances—in other words, triggering an allergic reaction. The allergic reaction then creates inflammation, which in turn leads to inflammatory skin conditions such as psoriasis and eczema. How can sarsaparilla help? Sarsaparilla contains steroidlike compounds that bind to gut endotoxins and prevent them from leaking out into the bloodstream. Considering how difficult it is to treat eczema and psoriasis, sarsaparilla is certainly worth a try. If you have these skin ailments, I also recommend that you add milk thistle to your antiallergy regimen (see page 87).

Possible Benefits

Reduces inflammation by controlling endotoxins.
Relieves psoriasis and eczema.

How to Use It

Take one (2,000 mg) capsule three times daily between meals when psoriasis or eczema flares up.

SELENIUM

Selenium is a mineral that is not produced by the body and must be obtained through food or supplements. It is found in garlic, onions, red grapes, broccoli, Brazil nuts, whole grains, and seafood. If you are allergic to one or more of these foods (nuts, grains, and seafood are common allergens), you may not be getting enough selenium in your diet. Why should you worry? Several studies have documented that asthmatics have low levels of selenium. A recent study published in the *American Journal of Respiratory and Critical Care Medicine* (December 2001) found that people who ate the most selenium-rich foods had the lowest risk of developing asthma. Selenium is not an antioxidant by itself, but it is essential for the production of several antioxidants, including glutathione, one of the most important antioxidants for both lung and liver health. Glutathione is also an anti-inflammatory, which can help reduce the complications associated with asthma, such as destruction of lung tissue. Is there any evidence that selenium supplements can help asthma patients? One small study showed that 100 mcg supplementation of selenium daily did improve asthma symptoms in six out of the eleven people in the study, as opposed to improvement in only one out of ten in the placebo group.

Selenium, one of the better-studied nutritional supplements, has a long list of documented side benefits. It is good for heart health. In fact, people who live in states with the lowest content of selenium in the soil are three times more likely to die of heart disease than people who live in states with selenium-rich soil. (The worst states for selenium include Connecticut, Illinois, Ohio, Oregon, Massachusetts, Rhode Island, New York, Pennsylvania, Indiana, Delaware, and the District of Columbia. Colorado Springs, Colorado, has the highest content of selenium in its soil). Studies have also shown that selenium may reduce the risk of several different types of cancer, notably lung, prostate, and colon.

Possible Benefits

Reduces risk of asthma.
Boosts glutathione levels.
Reduces inflammation.
Prevents heart disease and several forms of cancer.

How to Use It

Take one (200 mcg) tablet or capsule daily. Or look for an antioxidant formula containing the right amount of selenium. Do not exceed 400 mcg of selenium daily. High levels of selenium can be toxic.

STINGING NETTLES

As its name suggests, the stinging nettles plant *(Urtica dioica)* should be handled with care. The bristly hairs on the leaves are very sharp, and will pierce the skin if you touch them, injecting it with an irritant that can cause a rash. (As I learned when I studied herbology in pharmacy school, it hurts!) The good news is, an oral preparation made from stinging nettles can take the sting out of your allergy symptoms. The even better news is that you don't have to harvest this plant on your own anymore. You'll find easy-to-use capsules and extract at most natural food stores and pharmacies.

In one double blind, placebo-controlled study conducted during hay fever season (early May through early July) at the National College of Naturopathic Medicine in Portland, allergy sufferers were given either a placebo or freeze-dried nettles leaf capsules daily. Participants were told to take two (300 mg) capsules upon onset of hay fever symptoms, and then to wait an hour and assess their level of improvement. Of the people taking the stinging nettles, 58 percent rated the treatment as moderately or highly effective as opposed to 37 percent of those taking the placebo. Thirty-two percent of the stinging nettles users said they experienced *dramatic* improvement! This is not to suggest that stinging nettles is a cure for hay fever, but it appears that it can help reduce symptoms.

In rare cases, stinging nettles may cause an upset stomach, and it should always be taken with food. I think it works best when combined with other supplements, such as quercetin and vitamin C.

More good news about stinging nettles for men. Stinging nettles can inhibit the production of enzymes that contribute to enlargement of the prostate. In fact, it is a common ingredient in combination formulas for prostate health.

Stinging nettles is a natural diuretic that can literally wash the potassium out of your body. If you take stinging nettles, please be sure to replenish the lost potassium by eating a banana, or adding a few more servings of fresh fruits and vegetables.

Possible Benefits

May reduce hay fever symptoms.

How to Use It

Take one (300 mg) capsule with each meal, up to three capsules daily.

Caution

Do not use stinging nettles if you are pregnant or trying to conceive, or have kidney problems or heart disease.

SYNEPHRINE

Synephrine is an extract derived from immature bitter orange *(Citrus aurantium)*, or zhi shi as it is called in traditional Chinese medicine. Synephrine, a milder version of ephedrine from ephedra, is also used in herbal combination formulas to treat colds, flu, and asthma. If you're sensitive to stimulants in general and ephedrine in particular, you may also be sensitive to synephrine. Synephrine is a bronchodilator: It opens the bronchial passageways, making it easier to breathe. It is also a decongestant. Similar to ephedra, synephrine turns up metabolism and may facilitate weight loss.

Possible Benefits

Relieves congestion in nose and lungs.

How to Use It

Synephrine works best when combined with other herbs and supplements in antiallergy combination formulas.

Caution

Avoid products containing *Citrus aurantium* or synephrine if you have high blood pressure or heart disease. If you are sensitive to stimulants, synephrine could make you jumpy.

THYME

Extract of thyme *(Thymus vulgaris),* a popular herb used in cooking, is a traditional European remedy for coughs and bronchitis, inflammation of the bronchial tubes. As far back as the seventeenth century, renowned herbalist Nicholas Culpeper wrote that thyme is a "noble strengthener of the lungs." In fact, thyme is still used in commercial cough medicines in Europe and is now finding its way to natural food stores in the United States in combination antiallergy and anticold products. If you don't see thyme listed on the label, you may see one or both of its two volatile oils, thymol and carvacrol. These and other chemicals in thyme can soothe irritated bronchial tubes, thereby helping to control the urge to cough. They are also expectorants, which help clear the airways of excess mucus. Thyme is also a natural antiseptic and antifungal agent. Some natural healers believe that in many people, chronic yeast infections (candida albicans) may disrupt immune function and trigger allergic reactions. They prescribe natural antifungal agents such as thyme to control the yeast in order to restore normal immune function. If you have chronic yeast infections and suffer from allergy, you should talk to your physician or natural healer about taking steps to eradicate the yeast infection as part of your allergy treatment. Thyme is also included in many natural mouthwashes and toothpastes.

Possible Benefits

Relieves cough.
Antiyeast.
Bronchodilator.

How to Use It

If you have a dry, hacking cough, or bronchitis, look for thyme or thyme constituents in antiallergy products.

Thyme oil can be inhaled as a steam treatment for asthma or coughs.

Caution

Thyme oil, which is used in aromatherapy, should not be taken internally. In some people who have asthma, inhaling any substance with a strong odor may trigger an attack.

TYLOPHORA

Long used in the Ayurvedic traditional system of medicine from India, Tylophora *(Tylophora asthamatica)* is best known as a treatment for asthma and allergy. It is often included in special Ayurvedic antiallergy combination products that are growing in popularity in the West. Indian studies show that this herb is both an anti-inflammatory and an antihistamine and can reduce classic asthma symptoms such as shortness of breath and tightness in the chest. When Tylophora was tested against a placebo, patients reported a significant reduction in their asthma symptoms during the time they were taking the Tylophora as compared to when they were given a placebo. In this study, Tylophora increased the amount of oxygen in the lungs, improving lung capacity, but it did not achieve this in a subsequent study. In another study comparing Tylophora to standard antiasthma medications, this herb did not produce as good a reduction in symptoms as the drugs. This doesn't mean that Tylophora is not a useful therapy, but it does suggest that it is not for severe asthmatics (who should be closely monitored by their physicians). As with many traditional remedies for asthma, Tylophora may be best used as an adjuvant therapy along with conventional medicine to enable patients to use less drugs, or to keep symptoms at bay. Tylophora may cause temporary nausea and even vomiting in some people, and if you find you have unpleasant side effects that don't go away within a few days, discontinue use of this herb and try a different therapy. In my experience, however, most people using combination products with relatively small doses of Tylophora do not have any untoward side effects. The fresh herb and tincture are more likely to cause nausea than the dried powder, which is often put in capsules in combination with other antiallergy supplements such as boswellia and quercetin.

Possible Benefits

> Relieves asthma symptoms.
> Reduces allergy symptoms.

How to Use It

Look for antiallergy combination products containing Tylophora extract.

WILD CHERRY

For hundreds of years, herbalists have used a syrup made from the bark of the wild cherry tree *(Prunus serotina)* as a treatment for coughs due to bad colds, bronchitis, allergies, and even whooping cough before the days of the pertussis vaccination. To this day, wild cherry syrup is still widely used in popular brands of cough drops and cough syrups. It is also a common ingredient in cold and allergy products sold at natural food stores. How does it work? Wild cherry contains a muscle relaxant that helps soothe bronchial spasms. As you probably have noticed if you've used any of these products, the effect is almost immediate, but fairly short-lived. Nevertheless, in many cases, these products can provide relief from an irritating, hacking cough.

Possible Benefits

> Soothes bronchial passages.
> Relieves coughing.

How to Use It

Look for a natural cough syrup containing wild cherry. Take one teaspoon or use as directed.

YERBA SANTA

Yerba santa *(Eriodictyon californicum)* is a shrub native to the American West. Native Americans used it to treat respiratory infections, allergy, and asthma. It is an excellent expectorant. Yerba santa literally means "saint herb" in Spanish. It was so named by Spanish missionaries, who obviously held this herb in high esteem. Modern-day herbalists still do. Today, yerba santa is a common ingredient in antiallergy combination formulas.

Possible Benefits

Good for a bad cough.

How to Use It

Drink one cup of yerba santa tea daily, or find a combination antiallergy formula containing yerba santa.

ZINC

Last but not least is zinc, *the* mineral for immune health. Although zinc is not an antiallergy supplement in its own right, you can't have a well-functioning immune system without it. In fact, zinc lozenges are a popular remedy for the common cold! It doesn't cure the cold, but it does shorten its duration. The problem is, the typical, processed American diet is low in zinc, and many foods that are rich in zinc happen to be common allergens (such as seafood, eggs, wheat germ, and soy). Therefore, supplementation is often necessary. Zinc is also essential for the formation of many enzymes vital for normal body function, including the *super* antioxidant SOD (superoxide dismutase).

Possible Benefits

Boosts immune function.
Helps reduce the symptoms of the common cold.

How to Use It

Amino acid–chelated zinc and zinc piccolinate are the best forms of supplemental zinc. Take one (15–30 mg) tablet daily. If you are taking a multivitamin, it may include enough zinc. Easy does it! High levels of zinc can cause stomach upset.

CHAPTER 4

The Not-So-Great Outdoors

Hay Fever, Mold, Insect Bites and Stings,
Poison Ivy, Poison Oak, Poison Sumac,
Pollution, and Allergy-Free Sun Protection

HAY FEVER

You walk outside on the first beautiful spring day, take a deep breath, and then it hits you. You start to sneeze, your nose gets runny, your eyes get itchy and watery, your throat gets scratchy, and you feel miserable. You think you may have a cold, but your condition doesn't improve over the next few days—in fact, it gets worse. You develop an annoying postnasal drip and a hacking cough that keeps you up at night. Sound familiar? You've got the telltale signs of seasonal outdoor allergy, and depending on where you live and what you are allergic to, your symptoms could persist for weeks, months, or even all year long.

The popular names for your problem are rose fever or hay fever, depending on whether your symptoms are worse in the spring, when the roses bloom, or in fall, when hay is harvested. But in reality, your symptoms have little to do with either roses or hay. The true culprit is pollen. Pollen grains are produced by plants, trees, grasses, and weeds, as part of normal reproduction. They are so small that they are barely visible to the naked eye, but they are ubiquitous in the environment. When they become airborne, they can be carried by the wind for hundreds of miles. One plant can produce millions of pollen grains daily during pollination season. Some plants self-pollinate, that is, they can be fertilized by pollen from their own flowers. Others must cross-pollinate, that is, the pollen must be transferred from one plant to another to form the seeds that eventually bring forth new plants. Some of you may be thinking, "I thought bees took care of pollination." The fact is, insects pollinate only a small minority of plants, primarily the brilliantly colored flowers. The less attractive, run-of-the mill variety must fend for themselves.

'TIS THE SEASON FOR POLLEN

Typically, each plant has an annual pollinating period. Most pollination occurs during the warm months, from spring to fall. Since ice and snow stop pollen dead in its tracks, there is little activity during winter. Depending on where you live, the shorter the winter, the earlier the pollination season. Typically, trees pollinate first, grasses second, and weeds last, starting in late summer through early fall. The earlier the first freeze, the shorter the pollen season.

Has your hay fever been unusually bad in recent years? It's not your imagination. Due to changing weather conditions, experts predict that seasonal allergies are going to get worse. Global warming is producing shorter winters with less snow, which means that in many parts of the United States, the allergy season is getting longer.

Not all pollen is problematic—the heavier the pollen, the less likely it is to cause trouble. For example, pine trees produce a dense pollen that falls to the ground and does not typically become airborne. On the other hand, ragweed, a common weed in the eastern United States, produces a pollen that is very light and scatters easily, which makes it more likely it will land in your nose, or in your throat or eyes. It can travel for hundreds of miles in the wind! If you are allergic to pollen, it will enter your body via these pathways and trigger the production of histamine, which is the underlying cause of your symptoms.

During allergy season, the daily pollen count is often reported along with the weather. The pollen count is a rough measure of how much pollen is in the air. Obviously, the higher the count, the more likely people are to suffer allergic symptoms. The number reflects the grains of pollen per square meter of air collected over a twenty-four-hour period, but pollen counts can change rapidly due to wind and weather conditions. If you are highly allergic to pollen, pray for rain. Light rain literally washes pollen out of the sky, providing much-needed relief to allergy sufferers. Warm, breezy days are the worst because the pollen is carried by the wind.

If you have a pollen allergy, you could be sensitive to any number of trees, weeds, and grasses. Allergy testing can identify your specific allergens, which is useful if you are thinking of undergoing allergy shots. Because pollen is airborne, it is virtually impossible to avoid your allergen. Even if you kill all the weeds in your backyard, and eliminate the trees and grasses that are giving you problems, you still can't prevent pollen from traveling hundreds of miles from the originating plant and landing in your nose.

Following the right supplement regimen can help relieve allergic symptoms. The trick is to begin taking your supplements at least a month before your allergy begins. You can take a combination supplement specifically designed for seasonal allergies, or separate supplements.

Earl's Hay Fever Rescue Formula

I recommend using an antiallergy combination formula that contains:

MSM (1,000 mg)
Stinging nettles (300 mg)
Bromelain (100 mg)
Quercetin (400 mg)
Vitamin C citrus complex (500 mg)

Find a combination formula that contains these ingredients, or take each supplement separately *three times daily* with meals. Start taking your hay fever rescue formula at least one month before hay fever season. You can discontinue taking it after the first frost.

WHAT TO EAT DURING ALLERGY SEASON

Eliminating certain potentially irritating foods from your diet during allergy season may also help reduce symptoms.

For example, many allergy sufferers find that alcohol worsens their symptoms. In addition, if you are allergic to certain plants, there is a possibility that you may be allergic to fruits and vegetables that have similar proteins. This phenomenon is called cross-reaction. For example, people who are allergic to grass pollens may also develop allergies to tomato, melon, and watermelon. Those who are allergic to ragweed may also be allergic to bananas, melon, or honey. And people who are allergic to silver birch may develop allergies to apples, peaches, cherries, carrots, celery, and most nuts. Allergy testing can help identify potential problem foods. If you don't want to undergo allergy testing, but suspect certain foods may worsen your symptoms, keep careful track of what you eat. You can try the simple food elimination diet described on page 202 to keep track of which foods may be triggering symptoms. If your reactions to food are severe, or your allergic symptoms are worsening, please consult your physician immediately.

Try to eat a noninflammatory diet during your peak allergy season. Fill up your plate with fatty fish like sardines, salmon, and tuna (providing you're not allergic to them) and dress your salads with olive and canola oil, both of which contain essential fatty acids that soothe inflammation and promote healthy immune function. Avoid foods that are laden with saturated fat, such as red meat and full-fat dairy products—saturated fat promotes inflammation in the body, which may aggravate your allergy symptoms. In addition, fried foods and processed foods (packaged cakes, breads, and cereals) contain transfatty acids, which are also proinflammatory. Some studies suggest that a high-sugar diet, or a diet rich in refined carbohydrates (white, processed flour), can worsen allergy symptoms. So can too much caffeine. The fact is, it's important to pay attention to what you put on your plate all year long, but it's especially important to be mindful of your diet when your allergies are acting up.

Drink eight to ten glasses of pure, filtered water daily. Your body works best when it's hydrated.

There are other simple steps that you can take to reduce your symptoms and make your life easier during allergy season, as noted below.

• Keep pollen out of your home by shutting your windows and turning on the air-conditioning. Avoid window fans, as they pull outside air (which includes pollen) in.

• Do not keep plants indoors or have decorative floral arrangements indoors, fresh or dried.

• Pollen sticks to your clothing, so don't wear your outdoor clothes in the house. If possible, wash your clothes after wearing them outside.

• If you work around the yard, wear a mask that filters out pollen, dust, and mold.

• Shower after being outdoors to wash out the pollen. If you're up at night sneezing, try washing your hair before bedtime—it's a virtual pollen trap.

• Remember, the air is filled with the most pollen early in the morning and late afternoons on warm, windy sunny days. If your symptoms are bad, try to stay indoors during those times. Do outdoor activities in the midafternoon.

• Wear sunglasses outdoors, preferably the kind that wrap around the sides of your head. They not only protect your eyes against damaging UV rays, but can provide a physical barrier against airborne particles such as pollen.

• Avoid raking leaves—it sends pollen and other irritants into the air.

• Your car is not a haven from pollen! Roll up your car windows and turn on the AC (if you blow in fresh air, you will only add to your pollen woes).

• Even if you're not allergic to your pet, you could be allergic to the pollen that lands on his fur, and that he brings inside your house. So during allergy season, brush your pet outdoors, consider bathing him more often, and keep him off your bed and pillows.

• Time your vacation to avoid your worst pollen season and go someplace where you can avoid your particular offending plant. If you like the beach, it's a great vacation destination for allergy sufferers, since shore areas tend to be very low in pollen. If the mountains are more to your liking, the higher the better. There are few flowering plants at altitudes over five thousand feet above sea level, and therefore, there is likely to be less pollen. (Of course, if you get altitude sickness or respiratory problems, a high altitude may not the best choice for you.) A city vacation is better than a country vacation, but don't assume that you can avoid pollen altogether. There are parks in most cities, and many streets are tree-lined.

• Stress—both physical and emotional—can also make your allergy symptoms more severe. Be vigilant about getting enough sleep. A tired body is more likely to succumb to immune problems and more likely to pick up viral or bacterial infections, which can aggravate allergies.

Some people have tried to escape their allergies by moving thousands of miles away from the source. Unfortunately, it doesn't always work. First, people who are prone to plant allergies will eventually develop new allergies when they are exposed to new plants. Second, as the population becomes more mobile, the very plant you are escaping could pop up in any part of the country. For example, Arizona used to be a refuge for allergy sufferers because it did not have the same lush greenery as the Northeast. But as more and more retirees moved to that state from the Northeast, they often brought with them the same plants that they had in their yards back home, along with the offending pollen. When it comes to pollen, you can run but you can't hide!

Wash Out Your Eyes

If you have itchy, runny "allergic" eyes, try using an eyewash made out of the herb eyebright, which can relieve symptoms and reduce inflammation. There are several commercial products sold over the counter in natural food stores and pharmacies. I have found it to be helpful for allergic eyes. Here's another tried and true home remedy that I learned about from an ophthalmologist. Add one-quarter teaspoon of hypoallergenic, no-tears baby shampoo without conditioner to one cup of clean, warm water. Put a small amount of the solution on a clean washcloth and gently wash the inside and outside of your upper and lower eyelid. Do this every morning and every night, but use a clean, fresh washcloth each time. This simple wash is particularly good for people who tend to develop crusty mucous secretions on the upper eyelid. IF YOU

> HAVE ANY EYE INFLAMMATION, PUS, OOZING,
> OR ANY SIGNS OF CONJUNCTIVITIS, PLEASE
> CALL YOUR DOCTOR. YOU COULD HAVE AN
> EYE INFECTION.

OUTDOOR MOLD ALLERGIES

When you think of mold, you think of the icky stuff that grows on old bread or in the shower stall. Mold is not just an indoor problem (see Chapter 5, Allergy Proofing Your Home). The fact is, there are lots of mold spores flying around outdoors, and if you're allergic to mold, it can trigger the same symptoms as hay fever.

Mold is a member of the fungus family, and there are thousands of different types of mold in the environment. Fortunately, only a handful can cause allergic reactions in susceptible people. The most common molds in the United States are Alternaria and Cladosporium, which can be found both indoors and outdoors, but you may also be exposed to Aspergillus, Penicillium, and Rhizopus, among others.

Although both mold spores and pollen are carried through the air, there are significant differences between mold and pollen. First and foremost, mold thrives in warm, damp places. Rain makes mold worse. Furthermore, unlike pollen, some types of mold can survive freezing temperatures, which means that mold allergies can persist throughout the cold weather. During peak mold season, late July to late summer, when the weather is hot and humid, daily weather reports often include a mold count along with a pollen count.

Most mold allergies are not serious, but there are exceptions. For example, the Aspergillus mold can be particularly troublesome for people with asthma. It can lodge in the lungs, leading to a severe inflammatory asthma called allergic bronchopulmonary aspergillus. The symptoms include fever and coughing up of mucous plugs. If you have these symptoms, see your doctor immediately.

Some people with mold allergies find that their symptoms may worsen if they eat foods that are fermented with mold, such as soft cheeses like Brie or Camembert, or with yeast (another type of fungi). Mushrooms, vinegar, soy sauce, beer, and wine may exacerbate symptoms. Be vigilant about not eating old fruit that could be laden with mold, and don't keep leftovers too long in the refrigerator, as they are mold magnets.

If you have a mold allergy, be sure to keep your home scrupulously clean and try to make your backyard as inhospitable to mold as possible. Dead leaves should be cleaned frequently, since molds love rot. However, the job of cleanup is best left to someone who is not allergic to mold spores, since removing the leaves will send millions of mold spores into the air.

INSECT BITES AND BEE STINGS

For most people, a bee sting or spider or mosquito bite may be painful and annoying, but is not a serious health threat. The usual symptoms are localized pain, discomfort, and even swelling at the area of the sting or bite. Some people may even develop a mild allergy to the sting or bite—in which case, the swelling from an insect sting is a bit worse than normal, the mosquito bite turns into a red, angry welt. But for highly allergic people, bug stings and bites can be life-threatening.

Some two million Americans have allergies to stinging insects, such as bees, hornets, wasps, and fire ants. The allergy is not to the insect itself, but to the venom that is injected into the skin via the stinger. Mosquitoes, fleas, and other biting insects can deposit salivary gland secretions in the skin, which can also trigger an allergic response. In most cases, bug bite allergies tend to stay localized, whereas allergies to stinging insects are more serious. In the worst-case scenario, the allergic response is so severe, it spreads throughout the body, involving different organ systems. You may break out in hives—not just on the site of the bug sting or bite, but everywhere. In addition, you may have difficulty breathing, wheeze, feel abdominal cramps, feel cold, feel dizzy, have swelling in the lips, mouth, tongue, eyes, eyelids, palms, and soles of your feet, and may even lose consciousness. These are signs of anaphylactic shock, and if you have any of these symptoms, you need immediate medical attention. A half-million Americans have reactions to stings and bites that are so serious that they are treated in hospital emergency rooms, and sadly, up to 150 people die each year.

People who are aware of their insect allergies may carry epinephrine injections to prevent going into shock before they can get medical care. It's also a good idea to wear a medic alert tag that informs others of your allergy should you be unable to do so. Insect stings in particular can be so deadly that if you find that you have even a mild allergic reaction to a sting, tell your physician. The reaction to the next sting could be worse. Your doctor may decide to do further testing to determine how serious your allergy may be, to decide on the best course of action. In rare cases, some allergists may recommend immunotherapy (allergy shots) to desensitize people to insect venom, but there is always a risk that the treatment itself could trigger an allergic reaction. In most cases, if the allergy is deemed to be serious enough, your doctor will prescribe an epinephrine injection, which you will carry with you at all times.

If you are stung by a bee, wasp, or other stinging insect, and the stinger is still in the skin, remove it carefully. Flick it away with a knife or fingernail. Do not pull on it or you risk squeezing the stinger and spreading the venom throughout the bloodstream, which will only make your allergy worse. The goal is to keep the venom contained. Apply an ice pack to the sting or bite to reduce swelling and inflammation and limit the spread of venom. Don't apply the ice directly to the skin, it can cause further irritation. Instead, wrap the ice in a washcloth and leave the pack on the bite or sting for no more than twenty minutes every hour for the first six hours. If ice isn't available, wet a cloth in cold water and use that instead.

Do stay calm and don't run around a lot—it will only help spread the venom. If you've been stung on the arm or leg, you should initially *lower* the limb—it helps to prevent the venom from spreading. Later (I mean hours later), if you experience swelling, you can elevate the limb to reduce swelling.

If you are worried about developing an allergic reaction, although you have no history of it, you can take an antihistamine (such as Benadryl) to reduce your risk. But if there is any doubt in your mind about whether your reaction is normal, call your doctor, and if you have any untoward symptoms, go the nearest emergency room.

When it comes to insect stings and bug bites, avoidance is the best medicine. Although you can't always prevent them, you can make yourself a less attractive, and less accessible, target. Insect repellents, which I talk about later, work well for mosquitoes, ticks, and the like, but do not discourage most stinging insects. Stinging insects are typically attracted to bright-colored clothing (that look like flowers), food odors, perfumes, sugar, and even water. If you are in an area where there are stinging insects, wear drab colors, avoid eating outdoors, and don't wear fragrance or use scented skin creams. If you have a close encounter with a stinging insect, don't get him angry or frightened. Don't jump around or flail your arms, simply try to get out of his way as soon as possible. If you know that there is a nest of stinging insects in your backyard, call a bug control company, preferably one that uses natural methods. Remember, bees and wasps tend to nest beneath decks, or can lodge themselves inside any area where wires or pipes enter your home, or under wooden shingles.

In the case of mosquitoes and ticks, you have more to worry about than just an allergic reaction. Mosquitoes can spread West Nile Virus, a potentially fatal virus that until recently was only found in the Middle East and Africa, but has found its way to the United States. Since 1999, it has been responsible for nineteen human deaths, but it is particularly deadly to birds and horses. Ticks can spread Lyme disease, a bacterial infection that often begins with a rash and flulike symptoms, but if untreated, can lead to joint disease, heart problems, and serious neurological problems.

Mosquitoes and ticks will steer clear of insect repellent, but many people have reservations about using them. The most effective repellents contain the chemical DEET (n-diethyl-m-toluamide), which comes in a spray or lotion and can be applied directly to skin and clothing. However, DEET is a toxin, albeit a weak one, and some people (myself included) are concerned about the long-term health effects of using these products, especially on children. In some cases, allergic people may be allergic to chemicals in the insect repellent. If you live in a high-risk area that is loaded with ticks and mosquitoes, talk to your doctor about your options. There are some natural botanical products on the market. One product I like is Bite Blocker, a soy-based insecticide made by a company called Consep, in Bend, Oregon. You can use it on skin and clothing. Citronella lotion (also used in outdoor candles) is a time-honored bug repellent, but not as effective as those containing DEET, and many people don't like the odor. Some of the newer bug repellents contain eucalyptus and other natural chemical extracts that may work as well for many people, without the health concerns. (Of course, as I've said earlier, allergic people can be allergic to anything, so don't assume that if it's a natural product, it's safe for you.)

To keep mosquitoes and ticks at bay, put screens in all of your windows and make sure that there are no stagnant pools of water in your backyard that will attract bugs (for example, in a bird bath). Don't allow the grass on your lawn to get long—it provides a nesting ground for mosquitoes. Although they can be pricey, electronic bug zappers and coils may help reduce the bug population in small areas, such as your deck or backyard. However, in my experience, these products are not always effective, so don't assume that if you invest in one, your bug troubles are over.

When you go outdoors, cover up as much as possible. Wear a lightweight long-sleeved shirt and slacks instead of shorts and a tank top—smaller insects usually can't bite through clothing, although it may not deter a stinging insect. If you're hiking outdoors, wear cuffed pants that are tucked into your socks. Ticks in particular have a way of finding any opening! And do check yourself daily for tick bites. Remove any ticks that are lodged in your skin with sharp tweezers. You may have to look hard for them, as some are no bigger than a pencil dot. If you develop any unusual rash, get medical help immediately. Wear a hat— it protects you not only from the sun, but also from bug bites on your scalp. And never, never go barefoot. Everything from ticks to snakes to bees lurks in the grass on the ground.

If you get a mosquito bite, calamine lotion can help relieve the itch. (Don't use it if you're allergic to it!) Don't scratch! It will only make it worse and could cause an infection. If the itch is particularly annoying, try a low-dose hydrocortisone cream, but use it sparingly.

THE TRIPLE THREATS: POISON IVY, OAK, AND SUMAC

You don't have to be a woodsman to encounter one of these three well-known poison plants. In fact, in many parts of the United States, they can be growing right in your own backyard! And if you touch them, chances are that you will develop an extremely uncomfortable, itchy allergic rash.

Poison ivy, oak, and sumac belong to the Toxicoden-dron family of the Anacardiaceae species. The leaves, stems, and roots of these plants contain a chemical called urushiol, which is responsible for the nasty allergic response. You don't have to touch the plant directly to develop the rash; urushiol can stick to your clothes, garden tools, balls, or even your pets, and you can be infected by touching the "third-party" objects.

Within a day or two after exposure, the telltale rash begins as patches of red, itchy skin, but soon forms small blisters, which fill with a clear fluid. Eventually, the blisters break open and the rash disappears. In most cases, the rash is itchy and annoying, but not harmful, but in rare cases, it can be extremely painful, especially on particularly sensitive sites (such as the genitals), or can trigger a more serious systemic allergic reaction. If you develop a headache, or pain, or have fever or swelling, do call your doctor. The rash usually lasts about two weeks. If it lasts more than that, it could be something else, so have it looked at by a medical professional.

Scratching will not further spread the rash, but it can cause infection and further irritation, which is why it's not a good idea. Furthermore, the relief is short-lived—you're just itchy a few seconds later, anyway.

The problem with these poisonous plants is that the rash can be delayed by a day or two after contact, so you may not know when or where you were exposed. The sooner you find out the better. Since urushiol can remain on your clothing or shoes for up to a year, it's important to wash them off as soon as possible to avoid more exposure.

The best protection against poison plants is avoidance. If you garden, hike, or spend any time outdoors, you should know what these plants look like. Poison ivy has very shiny, reddish, orange-hued leaves. Both poison ivy and poison oak have a familiar three-leaf pattern, but poison sumac has paired pointed leaves. Sumac plants may also have greenish-white berries and are prevalent in the Southeast. Poison ivy tends to grow around lakes and streams in the East and Midwest, but can pop up anywhere. If you see anything resembling these plants, don't touch them.

If you garden, you may inadvertently disturb one of these plants. Try to minimize your risk of contact by wearing gloves and a long-sleeved shirt and slacks. Leave your gardening shoes outside your home and wash your clothes immediately after doing yard work.

If you find these plants in your yard, you should remove them, but do so carefully. You can remove them manually (wearing plastic gloves and a face mask) or use a weed killer. Don't burn the plants—the smoke can spread the urushiol and irritate your lungs. If you know that you've been exposed to one of these plants, clean the exposed area with rubbing alcohol *while you are still outdoors* so you don't spread the urushiol around your house. After you've cleansed with rubbing alcohol, rinse the area off with water before going indoors. Once inside, you can take a shower with soap and water, but don't use soap until you've removed the urushiol with alcohol or water, or you could just spread it around your body via the soap. Remember, you can re-expose yourself if you touch your clothes or shoes, so be sure to wash them down with rubbing alcohol and water before bringing them indoors. Better yet, throw them out! And be sure to throw out any work gloves that may have come in contact with the plants.

Calamine lotion, warm (not hot) Aveeno baths, or a bath with baking soda mixed in warm water are just some of the over-the-counter remedies that can help soothe the rash. Ask your doctor or your pharmacist for advice. Cool compresses soaked in Epsom salt water (use about two tablespoons of salt per cup of water) may relieve the itch. Over-the-counter corticosteroid steroids (Cortaid and Lanacort) can help relieve itching temporarily. Oral antihistamines may also help reduce itching, but do not use antihistamine creams on the rash, as it could cause further irritation. In severe cases, your physician may prescribe oral steroids. Steroids have their downside, and I certainly don't recommend that they be used routinely, but they may be necessary in some cases.

Woodsmen and herbalists claim that the plant jewelweed is an excellent treatment for urushiol-caused rashes. Herbalists have long used the leaves and juice of the jewelweed to treat this and other skin conditions. Jewelweed grows in the wild, often near poison ivy. True herbalists use the juice right from the stem of the plant. But if you're not up on your botany, you can buy jewelweed skin products specifically designed to treat poison ivy, oak, and sumac in natural food stores and on the Internet. Use as directed.

There are skin products on the market that claim to prevent urushiol rashes by providing a buffer between the offending substance and your skin. You can use these products if you like, and as long as they don't irritate your skin, but I wouldn't count on them to work all the time. You need to be vigilant about avoiding contact with these plants and take quick action if you should stumble upon them.

POLLUTION: EVERY BREATH YOU TAKE

Is the increase in air pollution caused primarily by the burning of fossil fuels responsible for the astronomical increase in the incidence of allergy and asthma? Most scientists agree that it's certainly a contributing factor, if not the major cause. Despite attempts to control pollution, it is still a major problem in most urban areas, from LA to Houston to New York, and even in some rural areas. According to a 2002 report issued by the American Lung Association (ALA), more than half of all Americans are breathing unhealthy air. The ALA blames the U.S. Environmental Protection Agency for not enforcing tougher air quality standards put in place in 1997 to reduce pollution across the country. In fact, a coalition of environmental groups are suing the EPA to get tougher with states and cities that are not complying with the law. So, what exactly is polluting the air? In particular, people are breathing unhealthy levels of two pollutants—ozone and soot.

First, let me clear up some confusion about ozone. Most of you have heard of the ozone layer, which is the protective layer of gas in the atmosphere that filters out ultraviolet rays from the sun. And most of you know that the ozone layer is disappearing due to pollution, and that this is causing concern among environmentalists. This not only contributes to global warming, but puts us at greater risk of developing skin cancer. So ozone isn't a bad thing, as long as it stays where it belongs.

The problem is, we are losing ozone where we need it, but we are being exposed to high levels of ozone where it doesn't belong—in our air. Ozone is released when sunlight hits the fumes emitted by the fuel-burning engines of diesel machinery, trucks, and cars. It is the primary ingredient in smog, the thick haze that plagues many cities during warm weather. Ozone is a powerful respiratory irritant that burns delicate lung tissue and can aggravate asthma and allergy. In many cities, ozone levels are tracked and reported on the news so that people with respiratory problems can try to avoid exposure on so-called "ozone alert" days.

But ozone is not the only thing in the air that's causing problems. Soot, or particulate matter, is as grave a danger. It can lodge deep inside the lungs, triggering asthma attacks, and is particularly dangerous to people with Chronic Obstructive Pulmonary Disease or emphysema. Pollution isn't good for anyone, but it poses a special threat to the elderly and children, who are most vulnerable.

How can you protect yourself against pollution? If you have serious respiratory problems and you're living in a severely polluted area (see the Terrible Ten list on page 135) you may consider moving to a part of the country where the air is fresher. (See the Let's Clear the Air list on page 135.) Of course, this advice may not practical for most people, who due to economic, family, or work attachments don't have the option of moving.

Your best defense is to be vigilant about monitoring the

air quality in your area and limiting your exposure outdoors on days when it is most polluted. In particular,
avoid outdoor exercise on hazy, smoggy days, especially
during the hours from 10:00 A.M. to 2:00 P.M., when the
air quality tends to be the worst. I'm not telling you to become a couch potato—you can still work out in an air-
conditioned gym, or run on an indoor, air-conditioned
track. But remember, when you exercise, you breathe in
more deeply, and you don't want to be inhaling dirty air
into your already irritated lungs and nasal passages. And of
course, roll up the windows in your car and turn on the
AC!

If you care about the environment, take a personal
stand by refusing to drive a gas guzzler. Drive only "clean,"
fuel-efficient cars, and consider carpooling whenever you
can.

For more information on lung disease, pollution, and
what you can do to help, check out the American Lung
Association website; www.lungusa.org.

Antioxidants Are Antipollution

People with chronic respiratory ailments such as
asthma have low levels of the antioxidant glutathione
in their lungs, which, among other things, helps to
detoxify harmful chemicals in the air that are inhaled
(such as ozone and soot). Take a combination of antioxidants, including vitamin C, vitamin E, NAC, selenium, and alpha lipoic acid, to boost glutathione
production and add to your defenses against pollution.

SUN PROTECTION

If you're prone to allergic dermatitis, summer can pose a particular dilemma. Should you wear sunscreen and risk a rash, or should you go without any sun protection and risk getting a sunburn, promoting skin aging, and even increasing the odds of developing skin cancer?

Although there are numerous sun protection products on the market that claim they are hypoallergenic, the fact is, people with truly sensitive skin may still find these products to be irritating. That a product is labeled hypoallergenic is no guarantee that you won't have an allergic reaction, all it means is that it is less likely to promote allergy. It is impossible to create a product that is 100 percent nonallergenic for everyone. However, there are things you can do to minimize your risk.

Ask your M.D. If you have highly allergic skin—that is, if your skin is irritated by most commercial skin products—ask your dermatologist to recommend a sunscreen. Some of the better products designed for supersensitive skin are only available through dermatologists or other health-care professionals.

Check your meds. If you are taking any medication, before going out in the sun, make sure that it does not cause photosensitivity. Many drugs increase your risk of sunburn or having an adverse reaction to the sun.

Look for purity. Buy colorless, odorless products.

Go PABA free. Use products that are PABA (para-aminobenzoic acid) free—PABA may be irritating to people with sensitive skin.

Don't overdo the SPF. Ideally, you should use a strong sunscreen, that is, one with a high SPF or sun protection factor, especially if you have fair skin. An SPF of thirty, for instance, means that if it normally takes you ten minutes to burn, when using the product, you can stay out in the sun up to thirty times longer without burning. (However, this is not a carte blanche to stay out in the sun. Even though you are not physically burning, UV rays are damaging the subcutaneous levels of skin.) The problem is, the higher the SPF, the more likely people with sensitive skin may develop an allergic reaction. So don't overdo it. Try a product with an SPF of fifteen, and do reapply often, especially after swimming. Even with sun protection, limit your sun exposure, especially during the peak ray hours of 10:00 A.M. to 3:00 P.M.

Consider using a sun block. A sun block actually forms a physical barrier between your skin and the sun's UV rays, and may be less irritating for some people than a sunscreen. Sun blocks contain micronized titanium dioxide. The problem is, they're more difficult to use and if not applied correctly, can form streaks on the skin.

Do a patch test. Before applying sunscreen or sun block to a sensitive area, such as your face, first test it on a small patch of skin on your upper arm. Apply a small amount of the product and cover it with a Band-Aid. Wait twenty-four hours. If there is no sign of irritation, you can use it on other parts of your body.

THE TERRIBLE TEN

According to the American Lung Association, these metropolitan areas consistently have the most unhealthy ozone levels in the United States.

1. Los Angeles–Riverside–Orange County, California
2. Bakersfield, California
3. Fresno, California
4. Visalia, Tulare, Porterville, California
5. Houston, Galveston, Brazoria, Texas
6. Atlanta, Georgia
7. Washington, D.C., Baltimore, Maryland
8. Charlotte, Gastonia–Rock Hill, North Carolina, South Carolina
9. Knoxville, Tennessee
10. Philadelphia, Pennsylvania, Wilmington, Delaware, Atlantic City, New Jersey—tied with Raleigh–Durham–Chapel Hill, North Carolina

LET'S CLEAR THE AIR

Want some clean air? Here are the metropolitan areas with the least ozone air pollution in the United States.

1. Bellingham, Washington
2. Colorado Springs, Colorado
3. Duluth, Minnesota, Superior, Wisconsin
4. Fargo, North Dakota, Moorhead, Minnesota
5. Flagstaff, Arizona
6. Honolulu, Hawaii
7. Laredo, Texas
8. Lincoln, Nebraska
9. McAllen–Edinburg–Mission, Texas
10. Salinas, California
11. Spokane, Washington

CHAPTER 5

Allergy Proofing Your Home

YOUR HOME IS SUPPOSED TO BE YOUR CASTLE, YOUR refuge from the perils of the outside world. You may be shocked to learn that if you have allergies or asthma, your home could be one of the most dangerous places on the planet!

Numerous allergens lurk inside the best of homes. Many of you are familiar with dust mites, molds, pet dander, and secondhand smoke as potential allergy and asthma triggers, but what you may not realize is that the air you breathe in your home may be even *more polluted* than the outside air. According to the Environmental Protection Agency (EPA), levels of pollutants can be two to five times higher indoors than they are outdoors. And like outdoor air pollution, indoor air pollution can also aggravate asthma and allergy symptoms in susceptible people. In fact, since you spend so much time in your home, indoor pollution can pose a greater hazard to your health and well-being than outdoor pollution.

Fortunately, there are simple and practical things we

can do to keep our homes as allergy-free and pollutant-free as possible and by doing so, reduce our allergy and asthma symptoms.

Before I go into detail about how to combat specific problems, I want to offer some general advice. When it comes to allergy proofing your home, vigilance is the key to success. You can never let your guard down. You need to establish a routine in which you continually keep such pests as dust mites, mold, and potential toxins under control. A word of caution: There are many antiallergy products on the market, notably chemical sprays and cleansers designed to kill household allergens such as mold and dust mites. Please use them sparingly, if at all. Many of these products contain powerful chemicals, and we do not know their long-term effects. They may prove to be perfectly safe, but many are untested. Remember, the goal of natural allergy control is to live in the *least toxic environment* possible. In most cases, a more aggressive approach to housekeeping will do the trick without declaring chemical warfare in your home. In fact, a recent study conducted by National Institute of Environmental Health scientists found that simple things, such as frequent washing of sheets in hot water and consistent vacuuming, significantly reduced allergens in the home. Sure, it may take a bit more work and planning than simply spraying some chemical around the house (which may or may not work), but in the end, the payoff is improved health and less need for "rescue medication" and its inevitable side effects.

DEFEATING THE MIGHTY DUST MITE

To allergy and asthma sufferers, dust mites are public enemy number one. These microscopic spiderlike creatures can trigger asthma and worsen existing asthma and allergic conditions. Dust mites are in virtually every household, but in varying degrees. Dust is not necessarily filled with dust mites—even if you have a dusty house, you may not have a dust mite–ridden house. Dust mites feed on dead human skin flakes, which are constantly being sloughed off to allow the growth of new cells. They also love mold. Dust mites thrive in humidity, so they are more prevalent in the rainy Northeast and Southeast than in the dry West.

The allergy is not to the dust mite itself, but to the feces of the dust mite, which can become airborne. The numbers involved in dust mite exposure are staggering. The average dust mite produces about twenty feces particles daily—the problem is, one gram of house dust contains thousands of dust mites. Decaying body parts of dead dust mites are also allergenic.

Dust mites pose a particular threat to asthmatics. About 10 percent of the general population are allergic to dust mites, but over 90 percent of asthmatics are allergic to them. When dust mites lodge in human lungs, the feces destroy sensitive lung tissue, which is what makes them so dangerous to asthmatics.

These little pests take root in mattresses, upholstered furniture, pillows, and carpets. If you are very allergic to dust mites, it's not advisable to do your own housekeeping. Every time you dust you are releasing dust mite particles into the air. If you have no choice in the matter, at least wear a face mask designed to screen microscopic particles such as dust mites. These masks cost a bit more than your standard dust mask sold at hardware stores, which can only screen out big particles. There are numerous brands on the market specifically designed for people with indoor and outdoor allergies. (If you have a latex allergy, make sure you buy a latex-free product.)

Protect your bedding. According to a national survey, an estimated 45 percent of American homes have enough dust mite allergen in their bedding to trigger an allergic reaction, and 22 million American homes have enough dust mite residue in blankets, pillows, and other bedding to trigger asthma attacks in susceptible people. This doesn't mean that Americans are necessarily bad housekeepers, only that dust mites are persistent. Keep in mind that you spend up to eight hours a day in your bed. Keeping your bedding as free of dust mites as possible will go a long way in helping to control your symptoms. Once again, there is no substitute for vigilance. Wash your sheets and pillowcases weekly, and your blankets every two weeks in *hot* water (at least 130 degrees). This will kill the dust mites and destroy the allergen. Use detergent designed for sensitive skin (that's for your protection, not theirs!).

Steer clear of "dust catchers" on your bed, such as frilly bed skirts, a fabric headboard, or your favorite stuffed animal. Avoid fuzzy blankets that attract dust.

Your mattress is a natural home to dust mites. At one time, your only option was to enclose your mattress and box spring in heavy vinyl covers, which could be uncomfortable, especially in warm weather. Fortunately, today, there are numerous companies selling excellent mattress and box spring covers made out of microfiber that help keep dust mites away from the mattress, but not at the price of comfort. They are a bit more expensive than standard mattress and box spring covers, but worth it. Be sure to buy a *zipper*-enclosed allergy proof mattress cover. For information on where to purchase these products, see Resources. If you have an old mattress that is already loaded with dust mites, it doesn't make much sense to use a protective covering. If you are allergic to dust mites, consider buying a new mattress and beginning your antiallergy regimen before your bed is invaded with dust mites.

Down with down! Don't use feather pillows or down comforters—they attract dust. Use only polyester-filled pillows and comforters. Primaloft, a synthetic down material, and Comforel are both excellent alternatives to feather pillows and comforters. Cover your pillows in a dust mite protective case similar to your mattress cover.

Keep your bedroom uncluttered. Do not allow dust to accumulate on surfaces. Piles of books, newspapers, and knickknacks attract dust. Clear wooden or lacquer surfaces are your best bet.

Avoid carpeting. Wall-to-wall carpeting can mean wall-to-wall dust mites. Stick to wood or vinyl floors and use washable area carpets if necessary.

Clear the air. A room cleaner with a HEPA filter (High Efficiency Particulate Air filter) can help reduce airborne dust mite matter as well as bacteria and viruses. The best ones are combination ionizers and air purifiers. There are many brands on the market but be sure to buy one with a HEPA filter. Maintain your air cleaner properly, and be scrupulous about following the manufacturer's advice to change the filter when needed. Also, be careful about maintaining your heating and air-conditioning units.

Change the filters often, and have the heating ducts cleaned routinely.

Window treatments. Avoid heavy draperies and curtains that collect dust. Instead, use wooden or vinyl shades or blinds.

Stuffed animals. Dust mites love these fuzzy friends. Wash stuffed animals in hot water once a week.

Overstuffed furniture. Upholstered furniture provides a wonderful home for dust mites. On the other hand, leather- and vinyl-covered furniture remains dust mite–free—they can't penetrate the outside covering. Dry steam cleaning can help reduce dust mites in furniture, but not entirely.

Your clothing. Dust mites can live on your clothing. Washing your clothes in hot water or dry cleaning them will kill dust mites and deactivate the allergen. What about your delicate items that cannot be washed in hot water? There are special detergents on the market that can kill dust mites in cold water—the downside is, they can be pricey, costing up to twenty dollars for a large container.

Vacuuming pros and cons. A standard vacuum can't effectively trap particles as small as dust mites. Very often, using a standard vacuum cleaner will simply blow around these tiny particles in the air, and in some cases, can be worse than not vacuuming at all. You have two options. You can purchase a special filter that goes into your existing vacuum cleaner that can help trap small particles such as dust mites and mold, or you can invest in a special vacuum cleaner designed to trap allergens, such as a Miele or a Nilfisk.

With the right equipment, vacuuming is an effective weapon in the war against dust mites. According to a recent study conducted at the National Jewish Medical and Research Center in Denver, a leading allergy research center, vacuuming daily with HEPA filters can significantly reduce allergen levels, which will, in turn, relieve symptoms. There are several brands of vacuum cleaners with HEPA filters on the market.

The right way to dust. When dusting, use a damp mop or cloth to trap more dust mites.

MOLD ALERT

Molds are microscopic members of the fungi family. There are thousands of different types of mold, and they are ubiquitous in the environment. Only a handful of molds are allergenic, and when these molds find their way into your house, they can cause real trouble for asthma and allergy sufferers.

The best way to protect yourself against mold overgrowth is to make your house as inhospitable as possible for these pesky microorganisms. Here are tips on how to prevent, hunt down, and rid your home of mold.

The bathroom. When it comes to mold, the bathroom is the most troublesome room in the house. Steamy showers and wet walls and floors attract mold like metal to magnets. Try to keep your bathroom as dry as possible. Immediately after showering, dry off the shower walls and floor. Invest in a high-efficiency exhaust fan for your bathroom, especially if you don't have a bathroom window. Clean your bathroom walls, shower stall, tub, and floor regularly. And don't forget the cabinets under the bathroom sink—wash them out thoroughly every few weeks, but leave the doors open so that they can dry. If you suspect mold is a problem, use a commercial cleanser that kills germs (it will also kill mold!) but beware of the fumes. Many household cleansers can be irritating to asthmatics. To reduce exposure, wear a protective mask over your nose that filters out chemicals. A diluted solution of chlorine bleach (one-half cup bleach to one gallon of water) is a terrific mold killer but can release chlorine gas, which may be harmful to asthmatics. I don't recommend that people with asthma use products containing chlorine. If you are allergic but not asthmatic, you may use these products, but only if your bathroom is well-ventilated. If bathroom tiles are already mold-infested, you may need to replace them and the drywall underneath.

Get rid of the bathroom carpet! It's a mold trap.

Latex paint is preferable to oil-based paint on bathroom walls. Some latex paints have mildew inhibitors, which will help prevent mold growth. Vinyl wallpaper and oil-based paint can hold water onto the surface of the wall, which may encourage mold to grow.

Use a specially treated mold resistant shower curtain and wash it frequently with soap and water.

Get a dehumidifier. Keep your indoor humidity level low, between 30 and 50 percent relative humidity. Use a hygrometer, which can be bought at most hardware stores, to keep track of your indoor humidity level. Humidity too high? Buy a dehumidifer for any potentially wet or humid areas in your home, including the basement or the laundry room.

Home humidifiers: Proceed with caution. If the air in your home is too dry, chances are that the heat is too high. Often, simply turning down the heat a few degrees will make the air less dry. If your nose and throat are still uncomfortably dry and you feel that you must use a humidifier, do not allow the relative humidity level to exceed 50 percent. Since humidifiers can also encourage the growth of bacteria and other microorganisms, clean out the humidifier daily (unplug before cleaning, of course!). Do not allow film and scale (a breeding ground for microorganisms) to develop. Be very careful that the area around the humidifier is not becoming wet, because that can encourage mold growth. Use bottled water specifically labeled "distilled" in your humidifier. This reduces the mineral residue, which could also be harmful. My best advice—use a humidifier only on days when you absolutely need to. Store your humidifier in a dry location when not using it. Be sure it's dry before you put it away and if possible, let it dry outdoors in the fresh air and sunlight.

Turn on the AC, shut the windows. In hot, humid weather, keep the windows closed and the AC on all day and night. Opening the windows at night or early in the morning when it's cooler only allows in moist air.

The bedroom. Don't keep laundry baskets or hampers of dirty laundry or wet towels in your bedroom, as they can attract mold and mildew. Don't keep plants in your bedroom, because the soil attracts mold. Throw out your old foam rubber pillows—they attract mold.

Carpet care. Steam-clean, don't shampoo your carpets. Steam-cleaned carpets dry faster and are less likely to promote mold growth. If an area of carpet becomes infested with mold, in many cases, normal cleaning will not work. Consider replacing the carpet.

Closets. Inspect the walls, floor, and ceiling of closets for mold growth. Periodically, open closet doors and air them out. *Do not put wet objects, such as damp rags or mops, in closets.* If you can, dry mops and rags out in the fresh air and sunlight.

The kitchen. Be sure your kitchen is well-ventilated and use an exhaust fan to remove cooking vapors. When boiling water, keep the lid on the pots to prevent moisture from escaping. Be vigilant about watching for plumbing leaks—even a few drops of water collecting under a kitchen sink can be an attractive breeding ground for mold. Dispose of the kitchen garbage daily—rotting fruits and vegetables encourage mold growth. Keep your refrigerator dry and clean—it's a likely site for mold growth. Don't allow food to get old and moldy in the refrigerator. Be vigilant about throwing food out before it goes bad.

The laundry room. Vent clothing dryers to the outside. Don't allow piles of wet laundry to accumulate. Dry wet clothing immediately after washing.

The basement. Dark and often humid, this room is a likely target for mold. Monitor your basement for signs of mold growth on the walls, floor, or ceiling, and if you do find mold, be sure to remove it immediately. Don't wait for problems—clean the floor and walls regularly. If you have a known mold allergy, do not attempt to clean the mold yourself because you will be exposed to high levels of spores.

Use HEPA filters. Use HEPA filters in your furnace; they filter out dirt and mold.

HEPA air cleaner. The same air cleaner that helps reduce dust mites and smoke can help clear the air of mold. It's a good idea to use an electronic air cleaner in the rooms in which you spend the most time, such as your bedroom or den.

Home maintenance. Keep your air-conditioners and furnaces cleaned and well-maintained. Change the filters often.

Serious mold infestation may require taking serious steps. There are environmental companies that specialize in mold removal, and in some cases, people may have to move out of their homes during the cleanup. Although this is rare, it is not unheard of. If you suspect you have a severe mold problem, your best bet is to contact your local EPA office for more information.

COCKROACH ALLERGIES

There are lots of reasons not to like cockroaches, but here's another. To many people, the feces and saliva of cockroaches are a potent allergen that can cause allergy symptoms or trigger an asthma attack. Urban areas and the southern United States are more prone to these pesky invaders than other parts of the country. Even if you have a clean house, you may still be at risk of cockroach infiltration. Cockroach eggs can enter your home on grocery bags or from a neighbor's apartment.

At the first cockroach sighting, you may be tempted to call in the exterminator, but keep in mind that pesticides are toxic not only to bugs, but also to humans and household pets, and may pose a particular risk to small children. Before trading one problem for another, there are some simple, safe, and natural things you can do discourage cockroaches from infesting your home. There are times, however, when you may need to turn to professional exterminators. Try to find one who understands your concerns and uses toxins sparingly, if at all.

If there's one, there are more. Complacency can lead to infestation. Don't assume that if you see just one roach, it's a lone straggler and there's nothing to worry about. Begin taking steps to prevent further infestation.

Starve them. Never ever leave food out. Store food in airtight containers and put leftovers away immediately. Wash dishes immediately after eating and keep your table and countertops clean and crumb-free. Like mold, roaches are attracted to warm, moist areas, so if your house is humid, be sure to read over my instructions on keeping mold at bay.

Keep your home clutter-free. Roaches hide in newspapers, boxes, and piles of junk. Make a roach homeless—throw out what you don't need!

Throw out the trash. Don't keep trash around the house, if you can help it. Use trash cans with tight lids, especially in the kitchen and bathroom. Throw out your trash daily, but if possible, throw out your kitchen trash after every meal.

Use natural methods. Before resorting to insecticides, try using boric acid (sprinkle boric acid on counters and in areas where you see roaches), poison baits, or roach traps. *Do not use boric acid near children or pets.* It can be toxic if ingested. Catnip is also a natural roach repellent. It contains the chemical nepetalactone, which sends bugs running. Herbalists recommend steeping catnip in hot water and, after the mixture cools, spraying it around areas trafficked by roaches. (Don't use catnip if you have a cat!) Most bugs, including roaches, are repelled by garlic. Leave peeled garlic cloves out on the kitchen counter to discourage roaches (and maybe anyone else who walks into the room!).

Spray carefully. If you absolutely must use an insecticide, never spray in areas where young children may inadvertently come in contact with the toxin—that is, where they play, crawl, or eat. When you spray, be sure that all food is put away, so there is no chance of its becoming tainted with the insecticide. Limit spraying to the infected areas; there's no need to spray all over the house.

Consider leaving. If your roach problem is so bad that you need to have several areas of your house sprayed, if possible, it's best not to be home during the spraying. Of course, you will need to delegate this task to someone you trust will not overspray or treat areas that you do not want treated.

Apartment dwellers. If your immediate neighbors are using insecticides, it could send the roaches running in your direction. If you must resort to insecticides, try to coordinate the spraying date with your neighbors. It's best to get professional exterminators to do the job. In the end, doing it right the first time may prevent future exposure.

INDOOR POLLUTION

If you think that exposure to dangerous chemicals is a problem solely of the workplace, think again. Millions of people are exposed to potentially hazardous chemicals in their own home, and to make matters worse, they are often completely unaware of the risk.

Indoor pollution can be caused by many things, from

fumes emitted by chemical cleansers to formaldehyde fumes seeping from pressed-wood products, including hardwood plywood and fiberboard, and even fumes emitted by new carpets. Indoor exposure to chemical toxins has been linked to numerous health problems, including sinus problems, throat irritation, headaches, dry eye, mental confusion, and chronic fatigue syndrome. Although these chemicals may not trigger the classic IgE allergic reaction (although in some people, they might), they may help set the stage for asthma and allergy down the road. How? Chronic exposure to chemicals can disrupt normal immune function, cause inflammation in delicate lung tissue, and create an environment in which allergy and asthma can take hold.

Some people are more sensitive to chemicals than others. In recent years, alternative physicians have identified a condition called multiple chemical sensitivity in which the affected individual suffers a wide range of symptoms— from allergy to headaches to fatigue to mental disorders— caused by constant exposure to toxins in food and the environment, even at low levels. Conventional medicine does not yet recognize multiple chemical sensitivity as a true diagnosis, but that's not surprising. It can take decades for an innovative concept to be embraced by mainstream physicians.

How do you know if your asthma or allergies are being aggravated by toxins in your home? When it comes to indoor pollution, newer homes may be more of a problem than older construction. For one thing, new construction may use synthetic building materials that are more likely to contain problem chemicals. Moreover, since the energy crisis of the late 1970s, building codes have been altered to reduce fresh air ventilation and promote energy conservation. These new "tight" buildings are more likely to hold on to chemical fumes and humidity than older structures, and therefore, put people at greater risk of developing health problems. This problem is so prevalent that it has a name—"sick building syndrome."

How is your home insulated? Injected, cavity wall insulation can pose a special problem because it constantly emits formaldehyde fumes, which have been linked to an increased risk of asthma in children. If you have a child with respiratory problems, it's best for him not to sleep in a room with this type of insulation, or you can have it removed from an existing room, and have the walls replaced. If you're concerned about toxins in your home—if you're wondering whether allergy symptoms or unexplained illnesses could be connected to chemical exposure—you can hire a building inspector to test for levels of particular chemical toxins. If you've been living in your home for some time, and you haven't had any health problems, there's no reason to panic, but if you're contemplating purchasing a new home, it certainly makes sense to check for potential toxins.

It may surprise you to learn that *you* may be responsible for many of the chemical pollutants in your home. For example, people with allergies or asthma should be careful about using aerosol cleaners, furniture polish, or air fresheners (aerosol or otherwise). Every time you spray, you get a lung full of chemicals. Furthermore, the toxins can linger in the air for others to breathe. As mentioned earlier, chlorine-based products can be irritating to asthmatics, and many people find ammonia is also irritating to the throat and respiratory system. Try to use nontoxic cleansers—Seventh Generation has a line of wonderful household products that are safer for humans and good for the environment. They are sold in most natural food stores and even some supermarkets.

If you use commercial cleansers, don't use more than one product at a time—combining chemicals can be dangerous. And be sure that your work area is well ventilated.

Paint and solvents can also be irritating to sensitive individuals. Fortunately, there are some brands of paint that are practically odorless and are least likely to cause problems in allergic people. For example, Benjamin Moore offers a nontoxic paint that is pure enough to be used in hospitals, but can also be used in homes. Even so, to minimize your exposure to fumes, save your painting projects and construction for warm weather when the paint will dry faster and you can open the windows or turn up the AC. Room air purifiers will help contain the paint odor. Wear a face mask that filters chemical particles during the painting or construction.

If you are having work done in your home, let your contractor know that you are concerned about chemical exposure and ask specific questions about the products he will be using on the job. Very sensitive people should consider leaving their homes during the construction period.

Your stove may also be a cause of indoor pollution. The burning of natural gas releases nitrogen dioxide, an odorless gas that appears to increase the risk of asthma and aggravate dust mite allergy. Studies show that teenage girls who are allergy prone may be particularly vulnerable to the respiratory effects of gas cooking. If you have a gas stove, invest in a powerful exhaust fan to clear the air.

SMOKING: PASSIVE AND ACTIVE

Tobacco smoke poses a particular risk to allergy and asthma sufferers and their families. Smoking increases the odds of developing respiratory problems, including asthma, emphysema, and COPD (Chronic Obstructive Pulmonary Disease), not to mention the fact that it is strongly associated with heart disease, diabetes, and many different forms of cancer. Each puff of smoke contains thousands of different free radicals that can overwhelm the body's antioxidant defense system. Smokers have lower levels of beneficial antioxidant vitamins C and E and glutathione, which protects the lungs. Every time you inhale, you are coating your throat, airways, and lungs with harmful toxins.

Despite the well-known health risks associated with smoking, there are 40 million smokers in the United States. What is particularly alarming about this statistic is that where there are smokers, there are people—often children—suffering the effects of secondhand smoke.

The EPA has classified secondhand smoke as a known carcinogen, which means that nonsmokers who may be exposed to someone else's cigarette smoke are at an increased risk of developing cancer, similar to the smoker. In fact, according to the EPA, so-called passive smoking is responsible for three thousand deaths from lung cancer each year.

Secondhand smoke poses a special risk to infants and young children, whose lungs are still developing. The EPA estimates that exposure to secondhand smoke is responsible for up to three hundred thousand respiratory tract infections in infants and children under the age of eighteen months each year. Up to fifteen thousand children will become so sick that they will require hospitalization. In addition, kids exposed to secondhand smoke have reduced lung function and are prone to ear infections. And here's a shocking statistic—according to the EPA, as many as 1 million asthmatic children have had their condition made worse by exposure to secondhand smoke. Even worse, exposure to smoke could trigger asthma in nonasthmatic children.

Pregnant women should not smoke nor be exposed to secondhand smoke—it can harm the developing fetus.

For the health of the family, it's imperative to live in a smoke-free environment. If a member of your household must smoke, let that person do it outdoors. And be sure that the people your children are spending time with, such as baby-sitters and day-care providers, are not smoking in their presence. (For information on smoke in the workplace, see Chapter 7.)

Allergy Proofing Your Car

You get into your car, roll up the windows, turn on the AC, and breathe a sigh of relief. You're thinking, "Aha! I've found a place where the allergens can't get me!" And you're wrong. The same allergens that are tormenting you daily have come along for the ride. A recent study published in the *Annals of Allergy, Asthma & Immunology* found that cars can contain significant amounts of dust mites and cat and dog allergen. And here's the kicker: The car owner doesn't even have to have a pet to be infested with pet allergen. How do allergens find their way into the car? Dust mites are brought into the car via your clothing, and then set up housekeeping in upholstered seat covers or in carpets. You can be exposed to pet allergens in any number of ways, including simply petting a neighbor's dog. The allergen clings to your clothing and gets on the seat of your car. So what's an allergy sufferer to do? Leather seats may help reduce the risk of dust mite contamination. In addition, you can purchase a portable air cleaner designed to remove allergens from your car. Be sure to buy one with a HEPA filter, as it can also help reduce pollutants that enter your car from other vehicles. Keep your car clean. Vacuum your car periodically with a vacuum equipped with a HEPA filter. Dry, steam cleaning of car upholstery can help reduce pet allergen and kill dust mites, and you may want to have your car thoroughly cleaned every few months. And be careful about replacing wet carpeting in your car, it could promote mold growth.

CHAPTER 6

Living with Pets

THERE ARE ABOUT *100 MILLION* PETS IN THE UNITED States and chances are, if you are reading this chapter, one or more of them live in your household. About 70 percent of all households in the United States have either a dog or a cat, but assorted birds, rodents (guinea pigs and gerbils), and even reptiles are also growing in popularity.

There are a lot of wonderful reasons to have a pet in your home. Pets provide their owners with companionship, friendship, and unconditional love. Numerous studies have documented that having a relationship with a pet can be beneficial to your health, from lowering elevated blood pressure to relieving loneliness and depression, especially among the elderly and homebound. And pets can teach children a great deal about responsibility and caring for others.

The problem is, about 20 percent of us are allergic to dogs or cats, and as many as half of us may develop an allergy to any kind of animal after exposure. Pet allergy can cause the same symptoms as pollen or dust mite allergy,

155

such as stuffy nose, watery eyes, sneezing, coughing, and wheezing, and can trigger asthma symptoms in susceptible people. Contact with saliva and dander can cause eczema or an allergic rash in some people. In many cases, pet allergy can be more severe than seasonal allergy, primarily because allergy season comes and goes, but your pet is with you day in day out, regardless of the season. So what's an allergic pet lover to do?

The first step is to understand what pet allergy is all about, so that you can determine the right pet policy for you and your family. In this chapter, I answer some of the most commonly asked questions about pet allergies and how to cope with them.

What is a pet allergy?

Contrary to common belief, people who are allergic to animals are not allergic to their fur, but to their dander, the small scales of skin shed by the animal, or airborne protein in the animal's saliva or urine. Although highly allergic people may have an allergic response to an animal outdoors, in most cases, indoor exposure is worse because the allergy is more intense. Cats are more likely to cause an allergic reaction than dogs because they are constantly preening themselves, thereby spreading saliva.

Another popular misconception is that short-haired animals are less allergenic than long-haired animals. This is not true: The length of an animal's hair has nothing to do with allergy.

Birds do not have saliva and have a different type of dander that tends to be less allergy-provoking. However, people can develop allergies to bird feathers and bird droppings, not to mention the fact that bird droppings can contain bacteria, fungi, and mold.

Every time you pet, or are licked by, an animal, you are exposed to potential allergens. However, you don't need to actually make physical contact with your pet to develop allergic symptoms. Dander and airborne protein from saliva can stick to upholstered furniture, get embedded in carpeting and bedding, even end up on the walls of your house. In other words, wherever your pet goes, allergens will follow.

In addition, furry animals can also attract dust mites, and if they go outdoors, can bring pollen and mold into your home.

How do you know if you're allergic to your pet?

It can take up to two years to develop an allergy to an animal after the initial exposure, more than enough time to get emotionally attached to your pet. If you suddenly develop persistent allergy symptoms, or if your existing allergies seem to be worse, it could be a sign that you are allergic to your pet. If you have other indoor allergies, however, it may be difficult to distinguish one allergy from the other. Skin testing against specific pet antigens can help further identify whether you are allergic to a particular animal. If you are not a pet owner, but find that you have an allergy attack every time you walk into the home of someone who has a cat or a dog, it's a safe assumption that you are allergic.

If you live with a pet, simply removing the animal for a few days to see if your symptoms subside will not work. It can take up to six months to fully rid a home of dander, and sometimes even longer.

Are there any completely hypoallergenic pets?

When it comes to allergy, it's impossible to say that anything is absolutely hypoallergenic, but reptiles and fish are considered the safest pets for allergy prone people. Although many of us would have trouble warming up to these cold-blooded critters, there are people who are as passionate about their pet snakes and tropical fish as others are about their pet dogs and cats. If you have a pet reptile, though, be vigilant about washing your hands after handling the animal to reduce your exposure to infectious microorganisms.

Dogs and Cats Can Have Allergies Too!

Your pet can be allergic to pollen and mold, just like you! If your pet is constantly sneezing, has a runny nose, or is itchy and uncomfortable, find a holistic vet who is knowledgeable in natural allergy relief. The itchier your pet, the more your pet scratches, and the more likely he is to deposit dander everywhere he goes. To prevent dry, sensitive skin, be sure your pet is getting enough essential fatty acids to both lubricate skin and control inflammation. Like humans, many pets are lacking these good fats. Simply add a teaspoon of flaxseed oil to your pet's meal once a day. Give your pet a daily multivitamin (there are several excellent brands for pets) to make sure he is getting enough A, E, and B, which are important to control allergy. During hay fever season, give your pet 1,000 mg MSM plus 500 mg vitamin C with flavonoids. You can

> mash the tablets up in his food. If your pet is over one
> hundred pounds, double the dose.

Do pets cause asthma in children?

This is an interesting question because the answer is not clear. Until recently, prospective parents with a family history of allergy or asthma were typically advised against getting a pet before the birth of their child on the assumption that exposure to the animal could trigger an allergic response that would spiral into asthma. Some went as far as to give away the family pet before bringing home the new baby! Now the experts aren't so sure if this was the best approach. Recent studies suggest that living with two or more dogs or cats during the first year of life may actually *protect* against allergy and asthma. Numerous other studies have documented that kids raised on farms, with intense exposure to a variety of animals, are less likely to develop asthma. Why? Allergy experts suspect that continuous exposure to high levels of animal dander and saliva may help desensitize the body to these allergens. On the other hand, low levels of exposure to animal allergens, such as encountering a pet for the first time at someone else's house, may trigger a strong allergic response. Based on these studies, no one is suggesting that parents of asthmatic children should fill the house with pets. Once a child has developed asthma, exposure to animal dander can induce an attack, and all potential allergy triggers should be avoided. However, there is little evidence that getting rid of the family pet before children are born will spare them allergy or asthma, and it may, in fact, increase the risk of their developing these problems. So the bottom line is, unless your doctor tells you otherwise, keeping the family pet is probably safe and will not cause a child to become asthmatic.

What if someone in your household becomes allergic to the family pet? Do you have to give your pet away?

This is another complicated question because it depends on a lot of different variables. On the one hand, a pet can become part of the family, and the prospect of giving up a beloved animal can be traumatic. On the other hand, you have to be concerned about the health and safety of your family member. If he or she is made severely sick by the pet, your only recourse may be to find the pet a new home. You need to make this decision with your family physician.

In some cases, if giving up the pet is not an option, the allergic person may have to resort to taking antihistamines or other medication, which may help to relieve symptoms. Immunotherapy or allergy shots are another option, but they can take up to three years to work, though many people feel some relief sooner. An antiallergy supplement regimen may help reduce sensitivity to allergens, but may not work against a strong pet allergy. Frankly, very little will.

If you live alone and are so allergic to your pet that physical contact is simply out of the question, I don't think it's fair to keep the animal. Animals need to be petted and loved, and if possible, should live with a person who can be affectionate.

If your family member's symptoms are not that serious, or your home is big enough to contain the pet in one area, you may have other options. Here are some tips on how to live with a pet in an allergic household.

Don't rub your eyes or face after handling your
pet. It can cause an allergic response in people who
normally are not irritated by pet allergen.

COEXISTING WITH YOUR PET

• If someone in your home is allergic to the family pet,
separation is the best policy: Set up specific "no pet zones"
in your home. Keep the pet out of the allergic person's
bedroom at all times. Keep the common areas of the home
(family room, dining room, bathrooms, and kitchen) pet
free. Remember, it's not just physical contact with the pet
that's problematic, but exposure to the dander and airborne proteins.

• If you have forced-air heating or air-conditioning, it
can carry the dander and other allergens throughout the
house. Put filters over your room vents or close the air
ducts in the allergic person's room. Use high-efficiency filters on the air-conditioning and heating system and
change them as directed.

• A room cleaner with a HEPA filter can help clear
dander from the room. Get separate room cleaners for
each room of the house.

• Wash down the walls of your home with a mild
tannic acid solution. It helps destroy dander. Tannic
acid is nontoxic but effective. Tannic acid products are
available in well-stocked pet supermarkets and on the
Internet.

• Use a vacuum with a HEPA filter. It helps control
microscopic airborne particles.

• Keep your pet off the upholstered furniture and carpeting. Wood and tile floors are better because they are less likely to be filled with dander. If keeping your pet off the furniture is not an option, put a protective cover over the furniture and wash it every few days.

• Set up a comfortable area for your pet with its own carpet and small blanket in a room where the pet is allowed.

• Do not use fabric drapes in the rooms frequented by pets—drapes absorb dander and pet allergen. Instead, use wooden or metal blinds.

• Have a nonallergic person in the household give your pet a weekly bath. Dogs may be less resistant to baths than cats. Get advice from your veterinarian about bathing a cat. You will have to wear gloves and protective clothing to avoid being scratched. Some manufacturers claim to have skin care products that reduce dander in animals—however, the effect is short-lived. Animals make dander continuously, so there is little respite.

• A well-cared-for, well-nourished animal will make less dander than a poorly nourished animal. Talk to your vet about feeding your pet the most nutritious diet possible.

• Keep litter boxes away from air vents that circulate air throughout the house. Be scrupulous about keeping litter boxes and cages clean. The allergic person should not do the cleanup!

If you have a severe pet allergy and are shopping for a new home, be sure to check whether pets have been living in a home before you buy or rent it. It can take months to completely rid a home of allergens, and you don't want any unpleasant surprises when you move in. If the house or apartment is covered in dander and pet allergen, it will require rigorous cleaning. You will probably need to change the carpet and wash down the walls.

CHAPTER 7

Allergies in the Workplace

YOU'RE BACK TO WORK AFTER A TWO-WEEK VACATION feeling healthy and reinvigorated, better than you've felt in months. But within a few hours, you've developed a stuffy nose and a dull headache, and you feel inexplicably tired. In fact, you feel almost as bad as you did before you went away. What happened?

You could be suffering from a workplace-related allergy. I know, we've all heard the old joke about being allergic to your job, but for millions of Americans, it's no laughing matter.

Occupational allergy is a growing problem in the Western world, in general, and the United States in particular. Over the past half-century, workers have been exposed to thousands of new chemicals on the job; about 250 of them have been documented to cause allergic responses in sensitive people. In addition, the same allergies that plague you at home—mold, dust mites, and even pollen—can make you miserable in the workplace. Poor ventilation in many of the newer office buildings is a major culprit. The

164

tight, energy-efficient buildings built after the 1970s energy crisis typically have windows that are sealed shut, which further compounds exposure to chemical fumes. In fact, in 1993, the EPA ranked poor indoor air quality as one of the top five environmental risks to human health.

Considering the fact that many of us spend nearly as much time at work as we do at home, a workplace allergy can have a detrimental effect on our health, well-being, and even our livelihood. In sum, if you don't feel well at work, you can't perform your best, and you can't enjoy your job.

Who is most likely to be affected by a workplace allergy? About 20 percent of the population is what allergists call clinically atopic, that is, they are more likely to react to potential allergens than others. If you have a personal or family history of allergy, you are also more likely to have workplace allergies. However, workplace allergy can happen to anyone, even people who never suffered from allergy before.

How do you know if you have a workplace allergy? Symptoms range from headaches to the standard allergic rhinitis to skin rashes to the life-threatening anaphylactic shock. Workplace allergy is also a major cause of asthma. In fact, according to the American College of Allergy, Asthma and Immunology (ACAAI), about 5 percent of all cases of adult asthma are work-related, defined as a "reversible obstruction of the airways, with its origin in the inhalation of ambient dusts, vapors, gases, and fumes that are manufactured or used by the workers, or are incidentally present in the workplace."

Some people may develop the telltale respiratory symptoms (wheezing, shortness of breath, chest tightness) or skin rashes shortly after exposure to a particular allergen, but others may not show symptoms until hours later. In some cases, it can take up to three years of exposure to a particular chemical to develop a full-blown allergic response. For example, many hairdressers develop an allergy to nickel, which is a common metal used in scissors. However, it often takes years for this allergy to surface.

How can you distinguish workplace allergies from other allergies? Generally, a workplace allergy improves when you're no longer exposed to the allergen, that is, on weekends away from the job or on vacations. Typically, these allergies worsen when you return to work.

Each occupation has its own particular allergy risks. For example, it's common for bakers to develop an allergy to cereal proteins or insect contaminants in food products or for food handlers to develop allergies to coffee beans or eggs. Hairdressers often become allergic to the chemical additives in shampoo and hair care products, and painters may become sensitized to the solvents in paints. Office workers may find they are allergic to ozone released by copy machines, or even the volatile organic compounds released by felt-tip pens. Not surprisingly, animal handlers often develop allergies to animal saliva and dander. Over the past two decades, millions of hospital workers have become allergic to one specific chemical—latex—which is used in the gloves medical workers wear to prevent the spread of infection, as well as in other hospital equipment. Latex is also found in countless household products and toys, which makes it extremely difficult to avoid (see Chapter 8, Allergy to Latex).

Given the vast quantity of chemicals in the workplace, there are numerous potential allergens. Sensitive people can have an allergic reaction to virtually anything from the cleaning supplies used by the maintenance staff to tidy up the office to the paint on the walls to the formaldehyde fumes emitted by the carpeting or office furniture. And if you're working in close quarters, the perfume or aftershave worn by a coworker can trigger an allergy attack. Some chemicals are more problematic than others. Diisocyanates (a class of chemicals widely used for coating and adhesives) are responsible for most of the new cases of occupational asthma, yet these chemicals are so ubiquitous in the environment that they're almost impossible to avoid.

Despite the vast number of allergens in the workplace, experts agree that it is possible to create a safe, healthy environment for workers. Here are some of the steps that employers and employees can take to maintain a work area that is as allergen-free as possible.

Eliminate allergens. If you develop asthma on the job, for your health and well-being, you must avoid the causative agent. When I was in pharmacy school, one of my fellow students suddenly developed hives, shortness of breath, and a drop in blood pressure during a laboratory class. He was in anaphylactic shock! It turned out that he was allergic to penicillin and was forced to switch majors. There was really nothing else he could do—handling these drugs was and still is an important part of a pharmacist's job. Depending on the workplace, an allergy doesn't necessarily mean that you will have to leave your job. Under the Americans with Disabilities Act, under certain circumstances, your employer may be required to accommodate your health needs, if possible. In some cases, your duties may be altered so that you are not exposed to the allergen. Sometimes, the solution is very simple. For example, hairdressers may become allergic to a particular chemical in shampoo, sodium lauryl sulfate. There are hair-care products on the market that don't contain this chemical that can be used instead. Or, if an office worker is allergic to a particular felt-tip marker, he or she should try a different brand of marker, which may not emit the same offensive fumes, and ask that others avoid using that marker when around them. If your allergy is not that serious, using a face mask to avoid fumes or using protective gloves (nonlatex) may do the trick.

Caution: If you suspect that you have asthma, you need to get appropriate medical attention. If you are at risk of anaphylactic shock and are working in an environment where there is even a remote possibility that you could be exposed to your allergen, you should have an emergency protocol in place at work. Make sure that your supervisor and coworkers know what to do and who to contact if you should have an attack.

Consider your allergies when choosing your job. Although you don't want your allergies to restrict your options in life, the fact is, if you have a tendency to be very allergic, it's wise to choose an occupation in which you are not constantly exposed to chemicals or allergens that could trigger an allergic response. For example, if you are allergic to household pets, veterinary medicine is definitely not for you! Or if you are highly sensitive to chemical fumes, painting and construction is a poor career choice. Remember, your health must always come first!

Better ventilation. Very often, simply improving the circulation of air throughout an office will help solve the problem. If possible, open the windows to let in fresh air.

If the windows are sealed shut, consider asking your employer to have new windows installed that can be opened. Be sure that the building staff is scrupulous about maintaining the heating and air-conditioning units, and that the system is cleaned frequently and that the filters are changed often. Use a room cleaner with a HEPA filter (High Efficiency Particulate Air filter) in your work space. It can help reduce airborne allergens near you, as well as dust mites, bacteria, and viruses. The best ones are combination ionizers and air purifiers. There are many brands on the market but be sure to buy one with a HEPA filter.

Move your work space. If you work near an area where there is more chemical exposure—for example, near a copy machine where you may be adversely affected by ozone emitted by the machine, or by chemicals used in toner—ask to have your desk moved.

Protective gear. If your work involves exposure to chemicals, be sure that your employer provides the correct protective gear, such as the right face mask, clothing, or gloves. Check with your union, OSHA, or human resources representative to make sure that you are being well protected.

Monitor the air. If you work in an environment in which you are routinely exposed to toxins on the job, make sure that the air is being monitored and periodically checked to ensure that you are not being overexposed.

Smoking policy. No smoking is the best smoking policy! Although many workplaces today are smoke-free, exposure to tobacco smoke can cause workplace allergies, as well as aggravate existing allergies. Due to the health threat that passive smoking poses to employees, it's imperative for companies to have a strict workplace smoking policy.

If smoking is allowed in the workplace, there should be a separate, well-ventilated area for smokers where the smoke does not contaminate the air of nonsmokers. It is not advisable to allow smoking in any work space where there is exposure to chemicals, such as nail salons, hairdressing salons, and factories.

Use nontoxic cleaning supplies. If you work in a closed office with poor ventilation, employers must be particularly careful about introducing unnecessary toxins into the workplace, such as harsh cleaning supplies. The cleaning crew should avoid using products with strong fumes. In addition, major work involving painting, renovation, or carpet cleaning should be done on the weekends to limit employee exposure to fumes.

The Cost of Allergies in the Workplace

It makes good economic sense for your employer to try to maintain an allergy-free work zone. Employee allergies are costing them money. Many employees are so bothered by allergy symptoms that they can't get enough sleep at night and are fatigued throughout the day. According to a study published in the *American Journal of Managed Care*, allergies resulted in a staggering $3.8 billion in lost productivity for workers. In addition, workers who take antihistamines that cause drowsiness may not be functioning at their best, and depending on their job, could be putting themselves and others at risk.

In fact, according to a clinical study conducted by the Group Health Cooperative of Puget Sound, people who use nonprescription sedating antihistamines are *50 percent more likely to have a work-related accident* than those who use natural remedies and nonsedating antihistamines.

CHAPTER 8

Allergy to Latex

LATEX IS THE NATURAL RUBBER MATERIAL MANUFACTURED from a milky fluid from the rubber tree, *Hevea brasiliensis*. (Although it may be called latex, products made of synthetic rubber are not really latex.) Allergy to latex was first identified in the 1970s, and it's estimated that up to 6 percent of the general population is allergic to specific proteins in natural rubber. The problem is far more prevalent among people in particular professions, especially health care workers. It wasn't until the late 1980s that latex allergy became a serious health hazard, affecting up to 12 percent of all health care workers. Why so many? In 1987, in response to the AIDS epidemic, the Centers for Disease Control recommended universal precautions to prevent the spread of HIV and hepatitis, which are carried in body fluids, such as blood. In record numbers, health care workers donned disposable latex gloves before handling patients, which were sprinkled with cornstarch to help make the gloves easy to slip on and off. What began as a method to protect health care workers and patients from infection turned into a nightmare for thousands of medical workers– doctors, dentists, nurses, and technicians. Between the years 1988–92, the FDA received more than 1,000 reports of serious adverse health effects from exposure to latex, primarily due to allergic reactions, resulting in 15 deaths. Even worse, the cornstarch in the gloves meant to make life easier for workers was actually helping to spread the latex allergen through the air.

The most common symptom of latex allergy is a skin rash on the area of contact, which can become quite severe, resembling poison ivy. Other symptoms include itching and swelling of the nose and mouth due to airborne latex particles spread by powder, and even asthma. There have been cases of anaphylactic shock due to latex exposure.

People who have medical conditions that require frequent tests or hospitalization are also at greater risk than the general public. In addition, latex is used in a wide variety of medical equipment, from air tubes to face masks, which can also affect patients. Children with spina bifida are at extremely high risk of latex allergy; about 40–60% of them will develop this allergy early in life.

But you don't have to be medical worker or a frequent patient to be exposed to latex. People who work in manufacturing plants that produce latex products are also at risk, and so are food handlers who routinely wear latex gloves. You can also be exposed to latex right in your own home or office. Latex is used in thousands of common items ranging from mouse pads to foam pillows to the soles of your shoes. The handle on the treadmill at the gym could be made of latex. The grip on your pen could be made of latex. Your bathing suit could contain latex around the waist for stretch. Your child's favorite rubber doll may contain latex. Even some brands of condoms and diaphragms contain latex, as do some sanitary pads.

Not everyone has to worry about avoiding latex products. If you're not exposed to latex routinely, and have not had a problem in the past, you probably don't have to concern yourself with latex exposure. (Of course, we know that when it comes to a condition like allergy, *never* use the word *never*—allergy prone people can develop a new allergy at any time.) However, do keep in mind that people with certain food allergies are more prone to react to latex than others. That's because of cross-reactivity, that is, the proteins that are causing the allergic reaction in latex are similar to the proteins in these foods. If you are allergic to bananas, avocados, or chestnuts, you are at highest risk of developing a latex allergy. If you are allergic to apple, carrot, celery, papaya, kiwi, potato, tomato, or melon, you have a moderate risk of being allergic to latex. Does this mean you need to avoid latex? If you are in the high risk group, I recommend exercising sensible caution. However, if you are in an occupation or a situation where you need to wear protective gloves, or are exposed to latex in other ways, I would seek out latex-free products and try to work in a latex-free environment.

Fortunately, hospitals have become more aware of the latex threat. Many have switched to non-latex gloves and equipment, although the switch has been slow because these products may cost more money. Some newer latex gloves have lower protein content than the old ones, and therefore, contain far less allergen. Powder is no longer used by most manufacturers. Some major medical centers have gone latex-free, although it's difficult to maintain an entirely latex-free environment. Visitors may inadvertently bring latex toys or toiletries, like a hairbrush or toothbrush with a latex handle, or even a balloon bouquet, to patients. If a hospital is still using latex, and many still are, workers or patients who have serious latex allergies may be transferred to latex-free zones within the hospital.

Interestingly, not all medical workers have been affected by latex equally. Although they used the same amount of latex, some hospitals had lower rates of allergic reactions than others. Why? According to a recent study, medical personnel who worked in a hospital with the best air circulation, that is, the freshest air, had half the amount of latex allergy reported as those who worked in a hospital that used recycled air. In other words, the better the ventilation, the cleaner the air, the less likely workers are to be affected by the allergen. I know I've said it before, but good ventilation is often the key to preventing allergy symptoms.

If you suspect that you have a latex allergy due to workplace exposure, report it to your employer. Depending on your industry, your employer may be required to report it to OSHA. Of course, seek medical help immediately, and make sure that you have an emergency protocol at work and at home.

If you have a latex allergy, avoiding the allergen is your best recourse. Here are some tips that will help you better cope with your allergy.

Medic Alert. Be sure to wear a medic alert bracelet stating that you are allergic to latex. If you should ever require medical assistance, you don't want to be inadvertently exposed to latex in the ambulance or hospital. If you have a severe latex allergy, be sure to alert your local hospital and ambulance company so that they send latex-free equipment in an emergency.

Check out products. Since so many products contain latex, if in doubt, call the manufacturer. Read product labels carefully. Avoid obvious rubber products, like rubberized bathroom carpets or rubber-gripped toothbrushes or latex mattresses. Many manufacturers are sensitive to the needs of latex allergic customers, and provide lists of latex-free products. Some products will actually say "latex-free" on the label. Beware the kitchen: Latex could be anywhere, from storage containers to rubberized sink mats and sink stoppers. Replace all rubber-gripped utensils with either wood, metal, or plastic.

Clothing. Anything with rubber could contain latex, from boots to bathing suits to swimming goggles. There are several clothing companies that cater to people with latex allergies. I will provide some names in the Resources section, but if you can, do a computer search on your own. Type in "latex-free clothing" on your favorite search engine (I use Google) and you'll be pleasantly surprised by the number of companies ready to serve you.

Latex-free office. Beware of rubber bands, pens, staplers with rubber bottoms, erasers, stamp pads, mouse pads, and anything that even *looks* like rubber. Fortunately, there are appropriate latex-free products that be used instead.

Toys. Children's toys are particularly perilous for the latex allergic—everything from dolls to rubber ducks to balls may contain latex. Some toy retailers, such as Toys R Us, have catalogues for special needs children that will specifically state whether a product is latex-free. Read the labels! If it contains latex or rubber, don't buy the toy. Once again, if in doubt, call the manufacturer.

The gym. Gym mats often contain latex, as do the handlebars on gym equipment. If you have serious latex allergy, the gym can be a dangerous place. I have not heard about a latex-free gym yet, but there may be some out there. Consider setting up a home gym, but do check with manufacturers about latex content before ordering any equipment.

Contraception. If you are allergic to latex, do not use latex condoms or diaphragms. Natural skin condoms are an option for men, but are not as effective against the spread of HIV and other sexually transmitted diseases. So-called female condoms made out of non-latex material are an option for women. Talk to your doctor about the best forms of contraception for you. By the way, some people first discover their latex allergy when they develop a rash or irritation after using a condom or diaphragm. If this has ever happened to you, tell your M.D.

CHAPTER 9

Protecting Your Skin, Nails, and Hair

SOME PEOPLE WEAR THEIR ALLERGIES ON THEIR SKIN—LIT-
erally. When these folks are exposed to allergens, they tend
to break out in rashes. Of all forms of allergy, this is the
most embarrassing, because it is the most difficult to hide,
not to mention the fact that in addition to being un-
sightly, allergic skin rashes can be very itchy and uncomfortable. They can also be unpredictable and hard to treat.
The key to maintaining healthy skin is to steer clear of the
allergens that are irritating your skin and triggering the
rash. I admit this is not always easy to do, but the more
you know about the relationship between allergy and your
skin, the better the odds of staying rash-free.

Many of you reading this chapter may have been diagnosed with *eczema,* the most common of all allergic skin
conditions. Eczema is also called atopic dermatitis, which
means inflamed skin. It is not contagious. The eczema
rash is characterized by dry, red, very itchy patches on the
skin. Itchy is the operative word—people with eczema can
be made miserable by the constant itch. Unfortunately,

scratching only makes the rash worse, causing the skin to get scaly and to thicken, and vulnerable to infection. Itchy blisters may form, which may burst on their own, or after scratching. Eczema can occur over a small part of your body, creating a minor nuisance, or over significant portions of your body, creating true misery. The rash most often occurs on the face, neck, and insides of the ankles, knees, and elbows, and on the hands, but it can pop up anywhere. Related rashes can also appear on the scalp.

Eczema may be confused with another common skin condition, psoriasis, characterized by the excessive production of cells of the outermost skin layers, which also produce red, patchy scales. Although the cause is unknown, psoriasis is believed to be autoimmune in nature, and may also be triggered by an allergen, infection, or stress. Although the two conditions may be similar, psoriasis lesions or plaques tend to look a bit different from eczema. They are generally redder and scalier, and are not necessarily itchy. About 10 percent of psoriasis sufferers also have related arthritis or gout, whereas neither condition is associated with eczema. In addition, psoriasis often affects the nails, causing ridges (see tips on nail care on page 189). However, most everything I recommend below for eczema will also be helpful to psoriasis sufferers, since both skin conditions can be triggered by similar irritants.

According to the American Academy of Dermatology, about 15 million people in the United States have eczema, which often strikes in early childhood. In fact, up to 20 percent of all infants have eczema, which many will outgrow by their teenage years. However, some people will have a tendency to develop eczema for the rest of their lives. There is no cure for eczema, but there are some effective treatments, and more important, strategies to help you control the rash, which I'll talk about later.

The million-dollar question is, what causes eczema? No one knows for sure, but there are some important clues. About half of all children with eczema have food allergies. In fact, eczema often first appears after the introduction of solid foods in infants. Eczema is also related to the immune system, which when exposed to an allergen or otherwise irritating substance goes into overdrive, triggering the inflammation on the skin, which causes the itching. In fact, eczema appears to run in allergic families—many people with eczema have other allergies, especially hay fever and asthma.

If you have a tendency to develop eczema, it can flare up at any time. It may be triggered by actual contact with a skin irritant, such as a soap, a cosmetic, a body lotion, or a detergent residue on clothing, or by nickel, a metal used in jewelry. Scratchy fabrics such as wool or chemical-laden synthetic fabrics may also cause skin irritation that can lead to eczema. It may worsen in dry, cold weather, especially if you have indoor heat turned up high. But your skin does not have to come in contact with an irritant to develop eczema. Eczema may also be caused by exposure to allergens such as animal dander or pollen, a food allergy, or a viral or bacterial infection that disrupts normal immune function, or aggravated by physical or emotional stress.

Standard treatments for eczema include oral antihistamines to treat the itching, corticosteroid creams in more severe cases, tar treatments, photo therapy (medically supervised use of sun lamps), and strong drugs to modulate the immune response. None of these treatments are cures, but they may help to control a flareup. The problem with a condition like eczema is that even when your skin is clear, there is no guarantee that it won't flare up again. That's why it's so important to adhere to a program to care for your skin and avoid the irritants that are most likely to cause problems. Here are some tips on how to treat a current eczema flareup, and more important, how to prevent the next one.

Deal with the itch. The standard advice to eczema sufferers is, "Don't scratch," because scratching worsens the rash. Of course, this is easier said than done. Scratching with your nails is particularly bad because it can break open the skin and promote infection. Instead, try gently (and I do mean gently) massaging the itchy area with the heel of your hand. If the itching is truly unbearable, talk to your doctor about using a mild hydrocortisone cream, but cortisone should only be used rarely, because it can become ineffective after long-term use, as well as thin the skin. Save this treatment for when and if you really need it. MSM therapeutic lotion, a natural and safe remedy, can be applied to the area up to three times daily. Cool compresses can help calm inflamed, itchy skin.

Keeping your skin well moisturized will help soothe itching. Avoid using standard soaps and body scrubs that dry your skin out, especially those that contain extra chemicals such as deodorants or bath oils that contain alcohol. If you have irritable skin, you never know what chemical will set it off! Only use special soaps specifically designed for allergic, dry skin. Aveeno and Basis are good cleansers that are usually not as irritating as standard soap. Aveeno oatmeal baths with added moisturizers are particularly soothing, but use them carefully, the tub can get very slippery. (Make sure that it's well washed out for the next person who uses it!) Soak in comfortably warm, but not hot, water for about fifteen minutes. Pat yourself dry with a soft towel—don't rub, it's too irritating. Use a moisturizer after your bath to seal in your natural oils. Curel, Lubriderm, and Eucerin are special moisturizers for people with very dry skin. Be sure to use unscented creams or lotions. If you live in a dry climate, or are exposed to indoor heat, remoisturize your skin at night or when it feels dry. If you prevent it from getting too dried out, you may prevent the start of the "itch."

There is a long tradition of using herbal skin care remedies for eczema. Some people get relief from skin lotions with chamomile, which can be purchased at natural food stores. Creams containing calendula and chickweed may also help soothe irritated skin. You may need to try several different treatments before finding one that works for you. Before using any skin product on large areas of skin—especially on eczema—do a patch test first. Place a small amount of cream or lotion on your upper arm and cover the area with a Band-Aid (latex-free). If there is no sign of irritation within twenty-four hours, try using the cream or lotion on a small patch of eczema. Wait for another twenty-four hours. If you see an improvement, you can use the product on other affected areas.

Be fussy about fabric. If you have a history of eczema, you must be very particular about what fabric you put next to your skin. Look for clothes made out of smooth, soft, natural fibers. Avoid rough, harsh fabrics and synthetic blends that may not allow the skin to breathe, capturing heat and sweat. Wool is tricky—if you are allergic to wool, even the softest wool may cause your skin to erupt. Even cashmere may be irritating to someone with a wool allergy, so do be careful. Sleep on natural, cotton sheets. The higher the thread count, the softer the sheet. If you have your sheets laundered out of your home, be sure that the laundry does not add starch, which stiffens the fabric. If your skin is very sensitive, consider wearing natural, organic cotton clothing. Some cotton cloth is now grown in shades of browns, reddish browns, and greens, which avoids chemical dyes. Granted, your color selection is limited, but if your goal is to avoid as many chemicals as possible, you can learn to like these natural cotton colors. There are several companies that sell nonirritating, natural clothing. For more information, see the Resources section.

Avoid tight-fitting clothing—especially clothing with tight, elastic waistbands. Any garment with rough edges that constantly rub against the skin can be very irritating, and could trigger a rash in susceptible people.

Beware of hidden irritants. Even if you are meticulous about the fabric that comes in contact with your body, if you don't wash your clothes and linens correctly, you could be inadvertently exposing yourself to unnecessary and potentially irritating chemicals. Many brands of detergent are filled with additives that could aggravate allergy prone skin, possibly triggering eczema. Therefore, try to choose brands that are designated hypoallergenic and are free of perfumes, dyes, bleaches, phosphates, enzymes, and fabric softeners, such as Tide Free, All Free and Clear, Woolite Hypo-Allergenic, Arm and Hammer Free, and Seventh Generation. In my home, we use a toxin-free all-natural orange cleansing agent in the washing machine, at the kitchen sink, and in all the bathrooms. It works great and it doesn't irritate our skin. It's also kind to the environment (see Resources). Measure detergent carefully—use only as directed. I always run the clothes through an extra rinse cycle to be extra sure that any soap residue is removed. If you have sensitive skin, it's a good idea to avoid fabric softeners.

Be vigilant about allergen control. Exposure to everyday allergens such as pollen or dust mites can trigger an eczema flareup in allergic people. If you have allergies and a tendency to develop eczema, be sure to read over Chapter 5, Allergy Proofing Your Home. In a recent study, the use of a mattress protector to control dust mites helped reduce eczema symptoms in allergic patients. If you have eczema, and you don't know the specific cause, have your doctor check you for common allergies, such as dust mites and pollen. If you test positive for a particular allergen, it's well worth the effort to avoid it. Pet owners, take note that animal dander and saliva can be irritating to your skin.

Watch your diet. Ask yourself, does your skin tend to worsen after eating a particular food? If you find that it does, it's easy enough to simply avoid the food or drink. It may not necessarily be an exotic food or drink—sometimes the most common foods or beverages turn out to be the culprits, such as your morning cup of coffee. Java addicts—take note. In one study, when heavy coffee drinkers cut out coffee, their eczema symptoms showed marked improvement. Switching to decaf won't do it. The allergy was to coffee, not caffeine. I gave up coffee years ago, and start my day with a bracing cup of green tea, which has a bit of a caffeine kick, but is a lot healthier than coffee. For more information on food allergies, turn to Chapter 10.

Stress reduction. If your skin is on edge, chances are, so is the rest of your body. Be sure that you are getting enough rest, and make time in your schedule to relax. Some of the ways people deal with stress, such as smoking and drinking alcohol, can actually aggravate eczema, and although they may provide instant relief, have negative long-term health effects.

SUPPLEMENTS THAT ARE GOOD FOR YOUR SKIN

Essential Fatty Acids

If you have dry, itchy skin, it's a sign that you are deficient in essential fatty acids. In fact, several studies have found that people with eczema and psoriasis do not process fatty acids normally. This problem is further compounded by a modern, overly processed diet that is sorely lacking in beneficial fatty acids, which only aggravates this metabolic glitch. Fortunately, there is compelling evidence that supplementing with essential fatty acids can help relieve some of the symptoms of eczema, notably the annoying itch. In one review article published in the *British Journal of Dermatology*, researchers analyzed nine placebo-controlled studies using essential fatty acids containing one in particular—gamma linolenic acid (GLA)—to treat eczema. The researchers found that most eczema sufferers benefited from the treatment, showing improvement in redness, scaling, and discomfort. Low doses of GLA were not effective; patients required at least 540 mg of GLA to get a good result. GLA is found in evening primrose oil and borage oil. It is also included in combination essential fatty acid formulas that contain other good fatty acids, including omega 3 fatty acids and DHA, docosahexaenoic acid, both of which are natural anti-inflammatories. Taking a combination essential fatty acid formula is useful because it helps relieve the inflammation that often accompanies allergy and is responsible for some of the nasty symptoms. However, if you take a combination formula, be sure that it includes enough GLA for your skin. In some cases, you'll have to take more capsules than recommended on the label to get your full 540 mg of GLA daily. Please keep in mind that some essential fatty acids, notably omega 3 fatty acids, are natural blood thinners. If you are taking medication to thin your blood, please check with your physician before using essential fatty acids. And if you are having surgery, tell your doctor that you are taking these supplements well before the surgery. They could interfere with blood clotting, and you may have to discontinue taking them a week or so before the procedure. In addition, the downside of fatty acids is that they can get oxidized or rancid (free radicals love fat!), so be sure to take your essential fatty acids with vitamin E and other antioxidants.

One interesting note: Evening primrose oil, which is rich in GLA, is a time-honored herbal remedy for infantile eczema.

Sarsaparilla

Sarsaparilla is a traditional herbal remedy for inflammatory skin conditions such as eczema and psoriasis. In fact, a 1942 study published in the *New England Journal of Medicine* reported a marked improvement in psoriasis patients who took a sarsaparilla compound. It works by controlling chemicals called endotoxins, by-products of bacteria that should be absorbed by the gut and sent to the liver for detoxification. People with both psoriasis and eczema often have higher-than-normal levels of endotoxins in their bloodstream. What does this have to do with their skin? Some researchers believe that endotoxins irritate the immune system, causing it to go into overdrive, creating an environment that promotes allergy and related conditions, such as psoriasis and eczema. Sarsaparilla binds to endotoxins, preventing them from entering the bloodstream and disrupting immune function. Take one (1,500–2,000 mg) capsule three times daily between meals.

Licorice Root

Licorice root, used externally or taken internally, is a traditional Chinese medicine for both eczema and psoriasis. Licorice is a natural anti-inflammatory, which helps explain why it would have a beneficial effect on allergy-related conditions. In particular, an ointment containing glycyrrhetinic acid, a constituent of licorice root, is used to relieve the itching and inflammation associated with both eczema and psoriasis. Studies have shown that this chemical works as well as hydrocortisone creams for inflammatory skin conditions. If you want to try this treatment, talk to your doctor. Since the cream is not sold in stores, you will need to have a special blend made for you by a compounding pharmacist.

Burdock

Similar to sarsaparilla, burdock *(Arctium lappa)* is known as a blood purifier that helps rid the body of toxins that could lead to other problems such as allergic reactions. Although burdock is a time-honored remedy for skin conditions such as eczema and psoriasis, there is little scientific research to validate its effectiveness. Recently, scientists have found that burdock contains compounds that are antibacterial and antifungal. What's interesting about this finding is that many researchers suspect that allergy itself may be triggered by a bacterial or fungal infection, and that these infections can cause flareups in conditions such as eczema and psoriasis. Therefore, burdock may actually help to treat these skin conditions by ridding the body of the problem that is causing them in the first place! Since burdock is nontoxic, there's no reason not to try it. However, pregnant women should avoid burdock since it may stimulate uterine contractions. Take up to three capsules daily.

Milk Thistle

Milk thistle *(Silybum marianum)* is best known as the herb for liver health, but natural healers often prescribe it for eczema and psoriasis. Here's why. As noted in the entries on sarsaparilla and burdock, several studies have found high levels of endotoxins circulating in the blood of people with psoriasis and eczema. (High levels of endotoxins have also been linked to arthritis and heart disease.) It's the job of the liver to detoxify poisons and prevent harmful substances from getting into the bloodstream, a conduit to the organs and tissues in the body. If the liver is not functioning at its peak, it may not perform its job as well as it should, allowing endotoxins to build up in the body, which could compromise immune function and lead to allergy. Take one (140 mg) capsule three times daily.

CARE OF YOUR HANDS AND NAILS

Your hands are the most hardworking part of your body, and the most vulnerable when it comes to skin problems such as eczema or contact dermatitis, caused by exposure to an irritant. No matter what your job, you can't help but come in contact with chemicals. Obviously, people such as medical workers, factory workers, beauty salon workers, and food workers handle chemicals daily, but even people in seemingly "nontoxic" occupations have their share of chemical exposure. For example, my friend, who is an attorney, developed a mysterious rash on her hands. It turned out that she was allergic to the toner used in photocopy machines, which came off on her hands when she handled photocopies of documents.

Homemakers are especially vulnerable to eczema because their hands are frequently in water while they are cooking or cleaning. In fact, "dishpan hands," characterized by red, sore, itchy patches on skin, is actually eczema.

If you have a tendency to develop eczema or atopic dermatitis, you need to be very careful about what you put on your hands. Wear soft cotton gloves when you do your housework or are likely to be handling potentially irritating materials (for example, when you're doing an art project with your child). Try to keep your hands out of water as much as possible. Scrape the plates clean (or wipe them with a paper towel) and put them in the dishwasher. Don't do hand laundry—use the hand laundry setting on your washing machine. If you must put your hands in water, wear protective gloves *(not latex!)*. Use protective cotton gloves and cover them with powder-free vinyl or neoprene gloves. You may even need to wear protective gloves while washing your hair, but be sure to use rubber bands around the edges of the gloves to prevent water from seeping in. If water gets into your gloves, take them off and dry your hands immediately and put on a new pair of gloves. Disposable vinyl gloves are best for handling food and can be purchased in many hardware stores or from catalogues.

Avoid using scented or antibacterial soaps on your hands (or anywhere else on your body, for that matter!). Wash your hands only when you need to, and use a gentle, nonsoap liquid cleanser such as Cetaphil. Pat your hands dry with a soft towel and apply a good moisturizer. Believe it or not, plain old petroleum jelly is great because it really locks in moisture and creates a protective barrier on your skin, but creams such as Curel, DML, and Vanicream are also good. Don't use premoistened wipes or antibacterial cleanser on your hands, as they could contain irritating chemicals. And don't use the harsh cleansers typically found in public bathrooms. Carry a small bottle of your own or just rinse well with water. Carry extra tissues with you so you don't have to use scratchy paper towels.

Rings can trap water and other irritants. Remove them before washing your hands or putting them in water.

If you have sensitive hands, chances are that you have

sensitive fingernails. Beware of using any strong chemicals on your nails. Some women may develop allergies to nail polish, nail polish remover, and the glue used to attach artificial fingernails. Even products that are supposed to be good for your nails, such as nail strengtheners, can trigger allergic reactions in susceptible people. In particular, nail products containing chemicals such as formaldehyde, methacrylates, and benzoyl peroxide may cause an allergic response. Not to mention the fact that if you have respiratory allergies or asthma, inhaling strong chemicals in nail salons may trigger an attack. If you have a history of peeling, splitting nails and suspect you are allergic to a nail product, try going without polish for a while and see if there's an improvement. If you go to a professional manicurist, select one whose salon is clean and well-ventilated. Make sure that the tools used by the manicurist are properly disinfected before use on each client, or even better, use your own manicure set to avoid infection. Always bring your own gentle skin cleanser and hand cream to make sure that you're not exposed to any irritants. Instead of ending the manicure with polish, have the manicurist gently buff the nails to a nice shine.

If you must wear artificial nails, be aware that a recent investigation by *20/20* newsmagazine found that some nail salons were using a potentially irritating chemical called methyl methacrylate (MMA), an inexpensive, fast-bonding adhesive, despite an FDA ban on the use of this chemical in nail products. The FDA recommends using another adhesive, ethyl methacrylate (EMA), which is less likely to cause an allergic reaction but is a bit pricier. How can a consumer tell which adhesive is being used? First, MMA has a very strong, bitter odor that can actually make

your eyes tear and can even make some people dizzy and
lightheaded. Second, since MMA is cheaper, the salons
using it tend to offer discount or very cheap acrylic nails.
If you see a price that seems too good to be true, it's a sign
that the salon is cutting corners, perhaps at your expense.
Third, if the manicurist is using a large brush to apply the
adhesive as opposed to a small brush, it's an indication
that she is using MMA as opposed to EMA. If in doubt,
ask the owner of the salon. Tell her that you have very sensitive skin and nails and will have a real problem if the
salon is using MMA. A smart salon owner will try to avoid
trouble, although there's no guarantee that you will get an
honest answer. If you develop any pain or discomfort after
having a manicure or getting artificial nails, be sure to see
your dermatologist immediately. Any yellowing or discol-
oration of your nail could be a sign of bacterial or fungal
infection and should be seen by your physician or natural
healer.

WHAT DOES HYPOALLERGENIC REALLY MEAN? (HINT: NOT MUCH!)

If you have a tendency to develop eczema or allergic dermatitis, chances are that you try to avoid putting potentially irritating chemicals on your skin by purchasing skin
care products and cosmetics that are labeled "hypoallergenic," "natural," or "fragrance-free." Unfortunately, these
words do not guarantee that you are buying a product that
will not irritate your skin. In fact, there is no such thing as
a truly hypoallergenic skin care product, because anyone
can develop an allergy to virtually anything. The term hy-

poallergenic suggests that a product is devoid of the usual chemicals that are most likely to trigger an allergic response. Since the FDA does not require manufacturers of cosmetics or other skin care products to substantiate their claims, you have to take their word for it.

The term natural usually means that a product contains botanical ingredients instead of man-made chemicals. However, bear in mind that pollen is a plant ingredient, and it causes lots of allergies. So, if you are allergic to pollen and other plants, you may want to avoid botanical products. And here's a real shocker—fragrance-free doesn't actually mean free of all fragrance. In fact, a fragrance may be added to a product to cover up the odor of another ingredient, and manufacturers do not have to list it on the label. Since fragrance is the most common cause of allergy in skin care products, the loophole in labeling can cause real problems.

To add to the confusion, the term alcohol-free doesn't guarantee that a product doesn't contain any alcohol, it only means that it doesn't have ethyl or grain alcohols. It could still contain fatty alcohols such as lanolin, a common irritant found in many moisturizers.

So what's a consumer to do? If you have very sensitive skin, you should stick to products developed by reputable manufacturers well-known for purity of ingredients, such as Clinique, Almay, and MD Formulations. Companies that stand by their products will let you return them, no questions asked, if they don't work for you. Always do a patch test before using a new skin care product—in fact, if in doubt, do it twice to make sure that it's safe. Ask your dermatologist for a product recommendation. In fact, today many dermatologists sell skin products formulated for sensitive skin that are not available in stores.

Be especially careful about applying any cream or cosmetic near your eyes without testing it first. The eyes and the skin around the eyes are particularly sensitive. Some women find that mascara that washes off with water and mild cleanser is less likely to cause irritation than waterproof mascara that is removed with special eye makeup remover.

People with sensitive skin need to be careful about using antiaging creams or products such as alpha hydroxy skin peels. Although these products are fine for most people, they can be irritating to people with highly sensitive skin. In addition, I don't recommend that people with highly sensitive skin undergo antiaging procedures, such as chemical skin peels or dermabrasion, unless they are performed by a dermatologist. These procedures erode the top layers of skin, revealing the more youthful skin underneath, and can be quite irritating if done incorrectly.

If you are in doubt about a product, call the manufacturer. Most of the good ones have their numbers printed on their labels and are eager to answer your questions.

ALLERGY TO JEWELRY

A friend of mine related the following experience, which I'd like to share with you here. On a whim, she had her ears pierced at a jewelry store at the local mall, but within a few days, the newly made holes became so inflamed and irritated that she had to take the earrings off and let the holes close up. A few weeks later, my friend put on a watch that she had not worn for a while, and much to her surprise, developed a rash on her wrist. When she went to her doctor, she found out that she was allergic to nickel, the metal used in her watch and most other inexpensive jewelry. But when she protested that she had worn that watch before and it never gave her any trouble, her doctor asked whether she had ever had her ears pierced. When she told him about her bad reaction to the ear piercing, she learned that the nickel in the earrings triggered an allergy to nickel, and for the rest of her life she would have to avoid wearing nickel next to her skin. This meant that she had to be careful about avoiding not only nickel-plated jewelry, but nickel-plated buttons on clothing or belt buckles. Even nickel-plated decoration on a handbag could cause irritation if it came in contact with her skin.

My friend's problem is hardly unique. Nickel allergy is one of the most common allergies, affecting up to 15 percent of the population. Most people are unaware of the allergy until they have their ears (or other body parts) pierced, introducing the nickel into the bloodstream, triggering the IgE antibody response. Although it is more rare, some people may develop a nickel allergy simply by wearing a piece of nickel-plated jewelry such as a watch or a necklace.

If you are allergic to nickel, it doesn't mean that you can't wear jewelry, but you do have to be careful about avoiding this offending metal. Since so many people are allergic to nickel, if you decide to get your ears pierced, it's advisable to avoid nickel-plated jewelry, especially nickel-plated posts that are inserted directly into the ear. Most people are not allergic to gold, platinum, or sterling silver jewelry. Surgical stainless-steel posts are also well-tolerated by most people.

Keep in mind that the strong antibacterial disinfectant typically used for several weeks after piercing (neomycin) may also produce an allergic response in some people. If you are allergic to neomycin, you can try using alcohol or hydrogen peroxide instead, but some people may also find these alternatives irritating.

Some manufacturers may advertise that they sell hypoallergenic jewelry, but in some cases, this may be a thin layer of gold plating over nickel, which could eventually erode. If you are allergic, be sure that you buy nickel-free jewelry. Beware of cheap jewelry, as it tends to have higher nickel content. Even if you're not allergic to nickel, wear nickel-free earrings only for the first six weeks after getting your ears pierced so that they can heal properly. Once the skin is healed, there is less chance that you will develop an adverse reaction to nickel. However, if you tend to be allergic and have irritable skin, I would advise not wearing nickel-plated jewelry at all.

Dark Circles under Your Eyes

Allergy sufferers often have dark circles under their eyes. It's not that their symptoms are keeping them up at night (although that could be the case). Chronic nasal congestion can increase the blood flow around the sinuses, creating more prominent blood vessels, thus making the under-eye area look darker. The problem is aggravated by the fact that the skin under the eyes tends to be thin and delicate, and thus, easy to see through. Getting your allergies under control may help reduce the dark circles. The best concealing agent is a sheer, hydrating cream that contains light-reflecting particles. A simple solution: If you are not allergic to Vaseline, try a thin film of Vaseline under the eye for a start. It's moisturizing and reflects light. Avoid using heavy, deeply colored coverups under the eyes, as they can actually call attention to your circles and make fine wrinkles more prominent.

CHAPTER 10

Food Allergy and Food Intolerance

DO YOU HAVE A FOOD ALLERGY? IF YOU'RE LIKE MOST people, you undoubtedly have a list of foods that may not agree with you, which has led you to believe that you are allergic to them. Although many people *think* they have food allergies, bona fide food allergy is relatively rare. In reality, only about 7 million Americans—2 percent of adults, and up to 8 percent of all children—have true food allergies.

What is a true food allergy? Similar to allergies to pollen or dust mites, food allergies are a result of an inappropriate response by the immune system. When you are exposed to the offending food, your immune system produces the allergy antibody IgE, which, in turn, stimulates the release of histamine by mast cells. Unlike environmental allergies, where the allergen enters your nose, or touches your skin, food allergies can be even more serious because as the food is digested, it reaches every point of your body.

Food allergy symptoms can vary from person to person depending on the severity of the allergy. Symptoms may be very mild—a slight rash, a few sneezes, and it's over—or very severe, even to the point of anaphylactic shock. Sometimes the allergy hits immediately, causing itching in the mouth or throat the instant you eat the offending food. Sometimes, it hits later. As food is being digested, new parts of the body are exposed to the allergen, triggering new symptoms such as vomiting, diarrhea, or stomach pain. As the processed food is absorbed into the body via the bloodstream, in severe cases, the allergen can cause a sudden drop in blood pressure. When the lungs are exposed to the allergen, it can cause respiratory symptoms such as sneezing or wheezing and even trigger an asthma attack. Finally, when the allergen is circulating throughout the body and reaches the skin, the allergic person may break out in hives or develop an eczema rash. Within a few minutes (or even hours) the symptoms tend to abate, and in most cases, you'll be fine. That is not the case, however, for severely allergic people, who can become violently ill, and in rare cases even die, from exposure to the allergen.

In cases of severe allergy, you may not even have to ingest the troublesome food to develop an allergic reaction. Simply eating a food that was cooked in the same pot as your allergen, or processed in the same food plant as your allergen, or came in contact with your allergen on a cutting board could trigger your allergy. This is called cross-contamination. Even inhaling fumes from an allergen could cause problems in highly allergic people. My point is, a serious food allergy should be treated as a potentially life-threatening medical condition. If you have a severe food allergy, you should be under the care and management of a knowledgeable physician or natural healer. You may need to carry an allergy kit (an epinephrine injection) with you at all times to treat yourself in an emergency. It is also important for you to become well-educated about food allergy and how to avoid your allergen.

FOOD INTOLERANCE

Countless people suffer from a different condition called food intolerance. When they eat a particular food, they may develop many of the same symptoms that characterize an allergic reaction, but do not have the actual IgE response. Food intolerance, however, can be every bit as serious as allergy, and can even cause a type of anaphylactic shock. Some foods are more likely to cause problems than others. For example, up to 50 million Americans are lactose intolerant—that is, they lack the enzyme needed to break down lactose, the predominant sugar in milk and other dairy products. When they consume dairy, they often suffer stomach upset similar to an allergy but do not produce antibodies against milk proteins, or have the other respiratory problems or hives typical of allergy. Many lactose-intolerant people, however, are able to consume dairy products that are lactose reduced, or can take supplements of the enzyme to aid digestion of lactose. A simple blood test can determine whether you are lactose intolerant. In contrast, people who are truly allergic to milk must avoid milk in all forms and may even react negatively to foods that contain even a small amount of milk protein.

Gluten intolerance (also called celiac disease) is another prime example of a condition that can mimic food allergy, but isn't an allergy. Gluten is a protein found in nearly all grains, including wheat, rye, and barley. When people with gluten intolerance eat products containing gluten, their immune cells target this protein as they would target an unfriendly virus or bacteria, creating an inflammatory response that can destroy the lining of the intestine, leading to serious malnourishment. The symptoms of gluten intolerance include many of the same GI symptoms associated with food allergy, but in fact, it's not a true allergy—it doesn't involve the classic IgE-mast-cell-histamine cascade typical of allergy. If you are gluten intolerant, your body produces a special antibody—the antigliadin antibody—which only targets gluten. If you are gluten intolerant, *any* grain with gluten will give you problems. Not so with allergy. If you are allergic to one kind of grain, such as wheat, you may be able to eat a different grain such as oats. (But do proceed with caution—in some cases, people who are allergic to one grain may also be allergic to others!) It is possible to be both allergic to wheat and gluten intolerant, and these people suffer terribly until they eliminate all gluten grains from their diet.

Many people develop intolerance to chemical additives in food, such as MSG, a spice used in Asian cuisines, or food dyes, but these are not necessarily true allergies. Nevertheless, they can cause discomfort and health problems.

Although there are significant differences between a food allergy and a food intolerance, there are also many similarities. Neither food allergy nor food intolerance is a good thing, and the best solution for both is avoidance of the food or food constituent that is causing your problem. (Although it may be useful in treating environmental allergies, such as an allergy to pollen, immunotherapy is not advised for food allergies.) Therefore, I am writing this chapter to help people with either problem—food allergy or food intolerance—learn how to manage their condition safely and effectively.

DIAGNOSING YOUR FOOD ALLERGY

How do you know which foods are causing you trouble? Sometimes, it's a no-brainer. For example, if you break out in hives every time you eat strawberries, it's a safe bet that you're allergic to strawberries.

Sometimes, the answer is not as clear-cut. For instance, if you are suffering general allergic symptoms, such as hives, stomach distress, or respiratory symptoms, and a food allergy is suspected, you may not know which particular food in your diet is the culprit. You cannot tell your doctor, "I think I have a food allergy," and expect your doctor to instantly know what food is causing you grief. You need to do a bit of detective work on your own. The first step is to keep an accurate food diary. Be as specific and detailed as possible:

- If you have an allergic reaction after eating, be sure to write down what you ate, when you ate it, where you ate it, and how long after eating you had the reaction.
- Did you eat anything that you may not have eaten before? Was the food prepared in a different way? Could the food have become cross-contaminated with something that you are allergic to?
- Did anyone else in your household or at the restaurant get sick? Unless you have the same allergy as

other family members, this could be an indication that the problem is related to tainted food as opposed to an allergy.

- Did you take an antihistamine? Did it help? Antihistamines will relieve hives caused by an allergic reaction.

- Did you eat before you exercised? Some people have allergic reactions to certain foods if they eat them before working out. But if you don't exercise after eating them, these foods don't cause a problem.

Even after taking a careful medical history, your doctor may need to use other types of allergy testing before determining you have a food allergy. Your doctor may recommend that you try the so-called elimination diet. It's simple to do, but it requires some patience. In the elimination diet, you eliminate a particular food from your diet for a period of two or three weeks to see if your symptoms go away. Then, preferably under your doctor's supervision, reintroduce the potentially offending food and see if your symptoms kick in again. If you develop allergy symptoms, it's a sign that you've targeted the right food. If you are prone to severe allergic reactions, that is, you are at risk of anaphylactic shock, or your system tends to react vigorously to allergens, you should not attempt to do the elimination diet unless it is under medical supervision. You could risk anaphylactic shock when you reintroduce the food.

The skin test is a standard way allergists determine whether you are allergic to a particular food. In the skin test, a tiny extract of the food allergen is either applied to a tiny scratch on your skin or injected into the top layer of skin, usually on the back or arm. If you are allergic to the substance, the exposed area will become red and irritated. However, the skin test is not always correct, especially if you have sensitive skin. You may have a positive skin test without ever having an allergic reaction to the food! The downside of the skin test is that it can cause a severe allergic response in highly sensitive people.

Blood tests such as the RAST and ELISA tests may measure the presence of food specific IgE in your blood, although even these tests are not absolutely definitive. The benefit of the blood test is that there is no risk of an adverse allergic response since you are not exposed to the allergen. In addition, one blood test can check for allergies for scores of foods, whereas the skin patch test can only check for one allergen at a time.

If you are unsure whether you are allergic to a particular food, let common sense be your guide. If you test positive for a particular allergen and feel better when you eliminate it from your diet, chances are you have a true allergy. Even if you don't test positive for an allergen, if a food doesn't agree with you, simply don't eat it. Be careful about eliminating too many foods from your diet—you don't want to cause nutritional deficiencies. If you are reacting negatively to a great many foods, you could have a digestive problem, and should consult your doctor.

THE USUAL SUSPECTS

The frustrating thing about allergy in general, and food allergy in particular, is that you can be allergic to virtually anything. Given the wide variety of foods eaten today, and the preponderance of chemical additives in the food supply, it seems that it would be impossible to pinpoint a particular allergen. The good news is that the overwhelming majority of food allergies in the Western world—more than 90 percent—are caused by seven common foods. The bad news is, as you will see from the list below, these are foods that are ubiquitous in the standard American diet.

Milk (cream, butter, dried milk powder, cottage cheese, yogurt)
Eggs (mayonnaise, meringue)
Soy (tofu, soy milk, tempeh)
Wheat (bread, wheat germ, wheat starch and flour)
Peanuts
Tree nuts (cashews, pecans, almonds, walnuts)
Fish and shellfish (shrimp, lobster, crab, saltwater or fresh fin fish, oysters, clams, scallops, mussels)

This doesn't mean that you could not be allergic to different foods, but if you are plagued with food allergy symptoms, consider one or more of these foods as possible culprits. It would seem obvious that if you're allergic to one of these foods, the best strategy is to simply avoid it. Unfortunately, that's easier said than done. Even if you are absolutely vigilant about avoiding your allergen, it may crop up in the most unlikely places in the most unlikely forms. For example, soy protein or wheat protein is often used as a filler for sausages or luncheon meats—and the label may simply say "texturized food protein." And there are numerous forms of milk by-products that are common ingredients in everything from waffles to cake mixes to so-called nondairy creamers. Unfortunately, the FDA allows food manufacturers to disguise their ingredients with hundreds of different chemical names that are unfamiliar to consumers. As of this writing, Congress and the FDA are trying to implement new regulations that would require food manufacturers to clearly list common allergens in easy-to-understand language, but little progress is being made. So, unless you know how to decode a food label (which I'll help you to do), you would never know that it contained soy or wheat or eggs or any other potential allergen.

If you eat in restaurants or at other people's homes, food can become cross-contaminated. In addition, creative chefs may add unexpected ingredients to their recipes. I remember one particularly heartbreaking incident in New York in which a young woman with a severe peanut allergy ordered a bowl of chili at a trendy restaurant and within minutes after eating it, died from anaphylactic shock. Unbeknownst to her, the chef had added a bit of peanut butter for flavoring! Who would have thought that a bowl of chili would contain peanuts? The moral is, if you have severe food allergy, you can never let your guard down.

Fresh, unprocessed food that you prepare in your own home will give you the least amount of trouble. It is less likely that there will be hidden chemicals or mystery ingredients in food in its natural state. Of course, many of us don't have the time or the inclination to cook everything from scratch, and we rely on commercially prepared food. In order to protect yourself against inadvertent exposure to your allergen, you need to become an educated consumer. In the sections to follow, I will give you information on how to cope with each of the common food allergies.

When in Doubt, Call the Manufacturer

Some, but not all, food manufacturers will state clearly on the label that their product may contain allergens or be processed in a plant where allergenic food is also processed. Many products, however, will simply list ingredients without stating this warning. Even if the food you are buying appears to be totally unrelated to your allergen, if you have a severe allergy to a common ingredient in food, I strongly recommend that you don't eat any processed food without first checking with the manufacturer. Be suspicious of a vaguely listed ingredient such as "natural flavorings." You want to know precisely what is in the product. Ask specific questions. For example, say, "I have a serious allergy to all tree nuts. Does your product contain any food by-product that contains nuts of any kind?" In addition, ask questions about potential cross-contamination. Was the food processed in a plant where the equipment was also used to process food that may contain your allergen? The major food manufacturers are receptive to your questions—that's why most of them display their phone numbers on the labels. They don't want people to have problems with their products. If you are not satisfied with the answer, don't buy the product.

If You Are Allergic to Milk

Avoid all forms of milk: This includes butter, artificial butter flavor, butter cream, cream, cottage cheese, dried milk powder, evaporated milk, all cheeses, custards, sour cream and sour cream solids, yogurt, ice cream and sherbets (sherbets often contain milk or cream, but natural fruit sorbets usually do not contain milk), and nondairy creamers containing milk solids. *Beware: Some brands of margarine contain milk solids.*

Breast milk is hypoallergenic: Infants who are allergic to cow's milk are not allergic to mother's milk, which is the best milk of all. However, babies can be exposed to a potential allergen from the mother's diet that finds its way into breast milk. Therefore, if family history suggests that an infant is going to be allergic to cow's milk or any other food, it's best if the mother eliminates the food from her diet while breast feeding.

Read labels: Milk or milk by-products are common ingredients in candy (particularly chocolate candy), baked goods, pudding mixes, and other processed foods. Even some brands of tuna contain casein, a milk protein, and chicken broth and soy cheese contain milk solids or milk by-products. Whey, another milk protein, is a common food ingredient that is also found in many protein powders and meal replacement energy bars. Sometimes the label will state clearly that a product contains milk or cream; sometimes it will not, and will use confusing chemical terms such as lactalbumin, lactalbumin phosphate, rennet casein, lactose, hydrolysates, and malt.

Milk substitutes: If you're not allergic to soy, soy milk is a good option. So is rice milk. Some natural healers tout goat's milk as an alternative to cow's milk, but in reality, it contains similar proteins and may trigger the same problems.

Nondairy isn't necessarily nondairy: Some nondairy

creamers and other products contain milk solids. Read the labels, and if you're unsure, call the manufacturer.

Lactose-reduced products won't work for allergies: Although sometimes promoted as "safe" for people who can't tolerate milk, lactose-reduced or no-lactose products are not any safer for people with milk allergies than regular milk products. These products, however, may be acceptable for people who are lactose intolerant. However, in cases of severe lactose intolerance, even a tiny amount of residual lactose may trigger an adverse reaction.

What about calcium? Dairy products are a good source of calcium, but not the only source. Canned salmon (only the kind with bones) is a great source of calcium. Green leafy vegetables, such as kale and broccoli, and calcium-enriched orange juice are good sources too. Calcium-enriched soy milk and rice milk are also excellent choices. To be on the safe side, you can also take a calcium supplement.

Acceptable milk substitutes: When baking, substitute equal amounts of water, soy milk, or juice in your recipes. Soy yogurt, made from soy milk, can be used as a substitute in recipes calling for sour cream or cream cheese.

Are kosher products okay? According to kosher dietary laws followed by religious Jews, eating milk products with meat products is a real No No. In fact, milk and meat foods are not supposed to come in contact with each other, requiring people who follow the kosher laws to keep separate "milk" and "meat" dishes and cookware. Therefore, kosher food is clearly labeled to alert consumers whether it is considered meat or dairy, or can be eaten with either milk or meat because it is a neutral food. First, the letter "K" or "U" tells consumers that a product is kosher. The additional letter "D" clearly states that a product contains milk or milk products; the letters "DE" mean that the product has been processed on equipment that also processes dairy products. Products labeled Parve or OU indicate that a product is milk free and meat free. However, according to Jewish dietary laws, a tiny amount of milk product due to accidental contamination (up to one-sixtieth part of the total food) is allowed in a Parve food, and although it may be a minute quantity, it could cause symptoms in someone with a severe milk allergy, but may be fine for someone with a mild allergy.

If you like to cook, kosher cookbooks provide a wonderful variety of dairy-free recipes and menus. Just be sure that you use milk-free ingredients.

Go vegetarian: Look for the "vegan" mark on food. It means that the product does not contain any animal products (such as milk) and is acceptable to strict vegetarians.

Medicine alert: Some drugs and vitamins contain lactose or casein as a filler, which may not be listed on the label. Don't take any medicine without first having your doctor or pharmacist check in the *Physicians' Desk Reference,* which includes a complete list of all ingredients. Use only brands of vitamins that clearly state "milk-free" on the label.

Eating Out

If you have a food allergy, be sure to tell the waiter about your allergy before ordering. Let him or her know, "I'm allergic to milk [or another food] and even small amounts of it can make me sick. I need to avoid food containing milk products, such as butter or cream, so before I order something, I need to know how it's prepared." If you have a serious allergy, consider calling the restaurant ahead of time and asking if it's possible to have the chef prepare a dish without your allergen. Many of the better restaurants will try to accommodate your needs. Do beware of the problem of cross-contamination. If you are so allergic to a food that even the tiniest exposure puts you at risk of anaphylactic shock, I would not advise eating out unless you are absolutely sure that you will not be exposed to your allergen. Depending on your food allergy, you may need to avoid certain restaurants altogether. For example, if you have a severe milk allergy, French cuisine, which relies heavily on butter and cream, may not be for you. If you have a peanut allergy, it's best to avoid Asian cuisines that use peanuts in food and peanut oil for frying, which may trigger an allergic response in some people. On the other hand, Asian cuisines tend not to use milk, which makes these restaurants a better choice for someone with a milk allergy.

If You Are Allergic to Eggs

An egg by any other name: Check food labels for egg additives. Eggs are used in products containing albumin (egg white), egg solids, egg substitutes (unless it specifies "egg-free"), mayonnaise, meringue, ovalbumin, eggnog, custards, and so forth. Be suspicious of any product beginning with the letters "ovo," which usually means it is derived from an egg product (such as ovomucin, ovomucoid, ovovitellin). Those catch-all ingredients "protein" and "natural flavoring" could mean that a product contains egg (and who knows what else!).

Where to look: Eggs or egg proteins are commonly used in baked goods, cake mixes, frozen foods, French toast, waffles, pretzels, muffins, and numerous recipes. It's a safe bet that any baked good that has shiny glaze has been brushed with egg. Most egg substitute products were not designed to accommodate the needs of people who are allergic to eggs: They are for people who need to cut back on fat and cholesterol. Therefore, many brands of egg substitutes contain egg whites, which are lower in fat and cholesterol than whole eggs, but are every bit as allergenic as egg yolks.

If you use canned soups or frozen dinners be aware that commercially prepared cooked pasta could contain egg or be exposed to egg products during processing. Fresh or dried authentic Italian pasta is usually egg-free, but read the ingredient labels carefully just to be sure. Prepared pasta dishes, such as lasagna, may include egg mixed with the cheese. Egg is often used in meatloaf and meatballs to bind the meat together. Even the white foam on latte could contain some egg, and so do some brands of ice cream. Remember, Caesar salad dressing often contains raw egg, although many chefs can do a terrific eggless Caesar. So before ordering any food outside your home, ask questions.

Vegan is good: Foods marked "vegan" are not supposed to contain eggs or any other animal product. Some brands of vegan lasagna are actually quite good and are made with soy products instead of eggs and dairy.

Tofu is a great substitute: Okay, tofu (bean curd) will never take the place of two beautifully poached eggs topped with Hollandaise sauce, but it can fill in for eggs in lots of other recipes. Try using mashed tofu instead of eggs in your favorite egg salad recipe. Be careful to use an egg-free mayonnaise. You will find several brands at most natural food stores. Soft tofu can be scrambled and made into an omelette.

Flu shots: The flu vaccine is grown on egg embryos and may not be appropriate for people with egg allergies. There does not appear to be a problem with other vaccines, however. If you have an egg allergy, check with your doctor before getting a flu shot.

If You Are Allergic to Soy

Rich in anticancer compounds, the soybean is one of the healthiest foods on the planet, but not for people who are allergic to it. Unfortunately, it's also one of the hardest foods to avoid. Soybeans are processed into dozens of products, from tofu (bean curd), to soy oil, to soy milk, to soy cheese, to soy flour, to imitation meat products. Soy protein is often added to processed foods to boost protein content. Soy is a common ingredient in commercial foods, ranging from commercial salad dressings, to frozen entrees, to sausage and luncheon meats, to broths and soups, to baked goods. Even your vitamin E capsule may contain some soy oil!

Hunting for soy: Once again, your only recourse is to read labels. Look for products containing hydrolyzed soy protein, lecithin (extracted from soy oil), miso (a salty condiment used to flavor broths and soups), vegetable oil (it could be soy), soy sauce, tempeh, texturized vegetable protein, natural flavoring, vegetable broth, vegetable gum, or vegetable starch. (Although some allergic people may be able to tolerate products with soy oil or lecithin, unless you are absolutely certain that these ingredients are safe for you, it's best to avoid them.)

Vegan is not for you: Many vegan products are rich in soy. Unless a product specifies it is soy-free, do not use it, and be sure to read ingredient labels carefully.

Watch out for other potential allergens: If you are allergic to soy, you may also be allergic to peanuts, green peas, chick peas, lima beans, rye flour, wheat flour, and barley flour.

If You Are Allergic to Wheat

Often called the "staff of life," wheat is a major component of the Western diet. It is also one of the most common allergens. Grains such as wheat are relatively new to the human diet and have been consumed for only the past ten thousand years. Many nutritionally oriented physicians believe that the human digestive system evolved on a grain-free diet, and that we were not designed to eat the quantity of grains that we eat today. In addition, the types of grains most people eat are made from processed, refined white flour, which does not contain any of the beneficial nutrients that are found in whole grains, such as bran and B vitamins. In fact, many nutritionists and forward-thinking physicians contend that a high-grain diet is the cause of many health problems today, from obesity to diabetes to heart disease.

Steer clear of all wheat: If you are allergic to wheat, you should avoid all forms of wheat, including whole grains. Unless you are committed to preparing your own food, this can be a monumental task. Like soy, wheat is morphed into dozens of different products and is frequently added to processed foods. It's obvious that the crust of a pizza is made of wheat flour, or that the bread on a sandwich is made of wheat, or that most baked goods are made with wheat flour. What you may not realize, however, is that the chicken cutlet on the sandwich has been coated in wheat bread crumbs (and even if it's not breaded, it could have been coated in wheat flour before it was sauteed), or that your favorite bottle of salad dressing could have added wheat protein as a thickener. Frozen and packaged convenience foods, such as waffles, pancakes, and French toast, are typically all made from wheat. Your favorite pasta is probably made out of wheat flour. The meatloaf at your local diner undoubtedly contains bread crumbs, and so do most brands of sausage. Even your bread-free, low-carb frozen dinner entree could contain some form of modified food starch made from wheat flour.

Read the labels: You will rarely see the word wheat on a label, but if you see the following ingredients, the product could contain some wheat: wheat bran, wheat germ, bread crumbs, bulgur, couscous, cracker meal, flour, high-gluten flour, high-protein flour, wheat gluten, wheat starch, soy sauce (contains wheat), starch, natural flavorings, graham flour, farina, cracker meal, hydrolyzed vegetable protein, vegetable gum, vegetable starch, semolina, pasta, and seitan.

Beware of new grains: In recent years, spelt and kamut, two alternative grains, have become popular. However, many people with wheat allergies could also be sensitive to these grains. On the other hand, buckwheat, also known as kasha, is usually fine as long as you do not mix it with pasta. This nutty-flavored grainlike food is actually not a grain, but a fruit. It is popular in Eastern Europe and parts of Asia, and is even gluten-free.

Go wheat-free: If you buy packaged food, assume that it contains some wheat products unless the label clearly states "wheat-free." This doesn't mean that you're never going to see another slice of bread or eat a waffle again. Many natural food stores and supermarkets now sell some terrific wheat-free, gluten-free products, from breads to bagels. For example, Vons offers a wheat-free, gluten-free frozen waffle that is quite delicious. You will find other brands of acceptable bread products on the shelves with the other baked goods or under refrigeration. Bread made entirely from rye flour is a good option, but some brands may also contain wheat flour. Read the labels or ask the baker. More good news: Rice and rice pasta are fine for people with both wheat allergy and gluten sensitivity, as long as they do not contain any wheat flour and are made solely with rice flour.

Do you react to other grains? People who are allergic to wheat may also be sensitive to other grains, such as barley, bulgur, and even oats. If you do eat grains, be on the alert for an allergic response. Don't gorge on grains—eating too much of any one food may also cause a food sensitivity.

If You Are Allergic to Peanuts

Despite their name, peanuts are not nuts, they are legumes, the food family that includes soybeans, lentils, kidney beans, and the like. Of all these foods, peanuts are the most allergenic, and the ones most likely to cause a severe allergic reaction, especially in children. The peanut allergen is so powerful that some allergic people will have a reaction if they are in the same room, on the same airplane, or even sitting in a ballpark where peanuts are eaten. In fact, even a small residue of peanut protein on a table, or a chair in a stadium, may be enough to trigger anaphylactic shock in highly sensitive people.

Given the fact that peanut allergy can be life-threatening, you would think that food manufacturers would go out of their way to clearly label foods containing peanuts. Not so! Peanuts are a common food ingredient and are frequently used in candies, ice cream, and cookies as flavoring. Even if a product does not contain peanuts, it could have been processed in a plant that also handles peanuts. So, if you are highly allergic to peanuts, you have to be extra-vigilant about avoiding contaminated food.

Baked goods can be a real problem. Recently, a manufacturer of a brand of chocolate chip cookies voluntarily recalled the product because it contained peanut flavoring that was not listed on the label, which caused several allergic reactions in unsuspecting consumers. I recommend that you check with the manufacturer before eating baked goods unless the package specifically states "no peanuts."

Watch Who You Kiss

According to a study published in the *New England Journal of Medicine*, peanut allergy can be triggered by kissing someone who has eaten peanuts. People with peanut allergies reported experiencing the telltale

itching, swelling, and wheezing after kissing a peanut
eater. At least one person had such a serious reaction that he had to be sent to the hospital.

Passed through breast milk: Doctors were mystified by
the fact that children with no known exposure to peanuts
in the past would suddenly develop a severe reaction the
first time they ate a peanut product. (Remember, with any
allergy, your body must first be exposed to the allergen before it can develop the antibodies that will attack it the
next time around.) As it turned out, these children had
been exposed to small quantities of peanuts in the past. If
a nursing mother eats peanut products, she can pass the
peanut protein on to her infant via her breast milk, possibly triggering an allergic reaction at subsequent exposures.

Read the labels: Avoid products containing peanut butter, cold-pressed peanut oil, mixed nuts, natural flavoring,
peanut flour, hydrolyzed plant protein, hydrolyzed vegetable protein, marzipan, or nougat. (Some studies suggest
that some people with peanut allergies can eat peanut oil,
not the cold-pressed variety. My advice: Check with your
allergist before eating any peanut product.)

Products to avoid: If you have a peanut allergy, avoid all
forms of artificial nuts, mixed bar nuts, and all candy unless you absolutely know that it is peanut-free and is safe
for you.

Eating out: Asian (Thai, Chinese, and Japanese) and
African cuisines may contain peanuts or use peanuts in
cooking. For example, Chinese chefs often seal egg rolls
with peanut butter. It's best to avoid these cuisines, or
cook peanut-free versions of these dishes at home. Beware
of chili! As noted earlier, some chefs add peanut butter as

a thickener. Before going to a restaurant, call ahead and make sure that there are peanut-free dishes for you.

Travel tips: In deference to allergic passengers, some airlines no longer serve mixed nuts on their flights. If even the smallest exposure to peanuts is a problem for you, call your airline ahead of time to make sure that the flight is peanut-free. Keep in mind, though, that you don't have control over whether or not other passengers bring a peanut food on board with them.

Are real nuts safe? Although peanuts are not tree nuts, most allergists advise patients who are allergic to peanuts to avoid tree nuts. Ditto for other nut butters, such as cashew butter. Since peanuts are often sold with other nuts, there is a strong chance of cross-contamination due to food processing. Apple butter is a great alternative for people who want a smooth spread but can't tolerate nuts.

Peanut-Free Ballparks

Thanks to the Food Allergy & Anaphylaxis Network, an advocacy and awareness group for parents with allergic children, some kids with severe peanut allergies can go to the ballgame. The group approached a local Connecticut baseball team and asked if they would be willing to set aside a food-free section that would be safe for allergic youngsters. The team owner agreed. Before the game, parents wash down the seats and railings of the special section to make sure that any peanut residue is eliminated, and special security is used to keep people with food and food vendors out of the allergy-free section. Similar food-free sections are being set up in stadiums across the country.

If You Are Allergic to Tree Nuts

If you have an allergy to tree nuts, you must not eat almonds, cashews, brazil nuts, chestnuts, hazelnuts, hickory-smoked nuts, pistachio nuts, walnuts, pine nuts, macadamia nuts, pecans—in sum, all tree nuts and nut butters are not for you. If you have a tree nut allergy, it's advisable to avoid peanuts, although unless you have a peanut allergy, you don't have to be as vigilant about avoiding even minute quantities of peanuts as those with bona fide allergies. Check with your allergist, but many people with nut allergies can tolerate coconut.

Nut oils: Use olive oil instead of nut oils. Avoid products that contain nut oils.

Baked goods and confections: If you have a sweet tooth, this is a difficult allergy. Nut extracts are a common flavor enhancer in baked goods, chocolate, candies, cookies, and ice cream. Products containing the elusive phrase "natural or artificial flavoring" could contain nut extract. Read the labels carefully and call the manufacturer if you are in doubt. Marzipan, a paste made out of almond, is commonly used in bakery cookies, so be sure to ask for an ingredient list before buying baked goods.

Eating out: Pesto sauce, a staple in Italian cuisine, is made with pine nuts, so if you eat in Italian restaurants, stick to red or cream sauces. (Nutmeg, a common condiment in cream sauce, is not a problem for people with nut allergies.) And remember that Waldorf salads contain walnuts and fish almondine is sauteed in almonds. Nuts can pop into the most unlikely recipes, so do ask your waiter before ordering a dish whether it contains nuts.

If You Are Allergic to Fish or Shellfish

Fish allergies can be quite serious, leading to anaphylactic shock in susceptible people. Therefore, avoiding your allergen is extremely important.

People who are allergic to fin fish may not be allergic to shellfish, and vice versa. However, if you are allergic to one kind of fin fish, such as sole, salmon, or tuna, chances are you are allergic to others. The conventional wisdom is to avoid them all. The same is true for other fish varieties. If you are allergic to crustaceans, such as shrimp or lobster, don't eat their close relative, crabs. And if you are allergic to a mollusk, such as oysters, avoid all others, including clams, mussels, and scallops. If you are very allergic to seafood, such as lobster, keep in mind that the protein can become airborne during cooking and trigger an allergic response. People with serious shellfish allergies should not attend shore dinners with steaming pots of lobster!

Fish products are less likely to be included in your favorite brands of baked goods or frozen food entrees (unless they are seafood entrees), so in many respects, this is a more manageable allergy than a wheat allergy.

No seafood restaurants: If you have a serious fish allergy, avoid seafood restaurants because of the risk of cross-contamination. Asian restaurants are also heavily into seafood and may not be the best choice for a person with a serious fish allergy.

Hold the anchovies: Anchovies are tiny sardines. If you're allergic to flat fish, do not eat anchovies on your pizza and order anchovy-free Caesar dressing.

Go vegan: Products labeled vegan should not contain any animal products, including fish or fish by-products.

Kosher means no shellfish: If you are allergic to shellfish, eat your fish meals at a kosher restaurant. All fish without fins (shellfish and mollusks) are forbidden under Jewish dietary law. Kosher frozen fish entrees are also fine for you.

Artificial seafood: Artificial crab meat may contain other types of crustaceans. Read the ingredient label or call the manufacturer to check before you eat it.

What about fish oil capsules? If you are allergic to fish, it's best that you get your omega 3 fatty acids from non-fish sources, such as flaxseed oil.

NOT AS COMMON, BUT JUST AS HARMFUL

If You Are Allergic to Sulfites

Sulfites are sulphur-based preservatives that are used to keep foods looking fresh, particularly fruits and vegetables, to prevent brown spots on commercial shrimp and lobster, to prevent the growth of bacteria in wine and beer during fermentation, and to bleach food starches. Sulfites are even used to maintain the stability and potency of some drugs. Although the FDA has classified sulfites as "generally recognized as safe," or GRAS, about 1 percent of the population is allergic to sulfites. People with asthma are at particular risk of having a serious allergic reaction to sulfites, which includes wheezing and difficulty breathing, as well as a headache. Therefore, asthmatics should not eat food with sulfites. Some researchers believe that a sulfite allergy may actually *trigger* asthma. Even though I'm not allergic to sulfites, I try to avoid all foods containing sulfites or other preservatives. In 1986, the FDA banned the use of sulfites on raw produce used in salad bars, a common source of exposure for unsuspecting consumers. Sulfites are still used in beer, wine, fruit and vegetable juices, canned vegetables, and many processed foods as a preservative. Prepeeled or precut potatoes (not fresh) may be sprayed with sulfites to prevent brown spots, and may be used to make hash browns or french fries in restaurants. (Order a fresh, baked potato instead.) Dried fruit is another leading source of sulfites.

Sulfites are listed on the labels of processed foods. Your best defense is to read the labels carefully. Avoid buying food in bulk (such as dried fruit) unless you know for certain that it is sulfite-free. Many natural food stores offer sulfite-free brands, but don't take the store's word for it, ask to see the original label on the package. If you eat shrimp or lobster, be sure that it does not contain sulfites. If you're buying it yourself, ask at the fish market. Some natural food stores offer sulfite-free seafood. If you're eating out, ask the chef. If you don't get a definite answer, order something else. By the way, having a sulfite allergy doesn't mean that you can't imbibe—I recently sampled a brand of organic, sulfite-free wine that was quite delicious. A well-stocked liquor store should have some sulfite-free products.

If You Are Allergic to Corn

Corn allergy is not as common as allergy to the other foods discussed in this chapter, but when it strikes, it can be severe. Furthermore, corn may be the most difficult of all foods to avoid. Why? I'm not just talking about corn on the cob, cornflakes, or corn chips. Most processed foods—from cereal to tomato sauce to soda to frozen french fries—contain some form of corn syrup or cornstarch. In fact, corn syrup is probably the most commonly used sweetener in the United States. To compound the problem, cornstarch and corn derivatives are used as thickening agents in countless foods. If you are allergic to corn, you will probably have to avoid all processed foods and beverages, unless you know for sure that they do not contain corn. Once you begin reading ingredient labels, you will be astonished at the unlikely places corn products show up. Ingredients such as dextrose, maltodextrin, high-fructose corn syrup, modified food starch, baking powder, caramel, syrup, natural flavoring, and natural sweeteners could mean a product contains corn. Corn products may also be used in drugs, vitamins, skin care products, and body powders. There are so many different corn-derived food additives that if you have a serious corn allergy, I strongly urge you to call the manufacturer before eating a processed food product. Keep in mind that manufacturers often change their ingredients, so always read the label before consuming a product, even if you believe it to be safe. Although many people with corn allergy can tolerate corn oil, those with severe allergy to corn may not be able to. If you have a corn allergy, I recommend working with a knowledgeable physician and dietitian to help you devise the right eating plan for you.

Don't despair if you have a sweet tooth—corn is not the only sweetener in town. If you are allergic to corn, you can safely use other sweeteners such as fruit juice, honey, beet cane sugar, and 100 percent natural maple syrup. If you cook, use rice starch and potato starch instead of cornstarch as a thickening agent, and for baking, baking soda and cream of tartar are safe leavening agents.

TIPS FOR PARENTS OF ALLERGIC CHILDREN

As the father of an allergic child, I know how difficult it can be to tell your child he or she can't risk eating the birthday cake at a classmate's party or even a casual snack served at a friend's house. At best, it makes a child feel self-conscious, and at worst, people think that you are an ogre trying to take the fun out of childhood. You live in fear that "well-meaning" friends and caregivers may even try to sneak your child snacks on the side, assuming that you are being overprotective. I have found, however, that once you educate people about allergy, they will better understand your fears and will be more likely to comply with your child's food restrictions. Here are some tips that can help the parents of allergic children better cope with their children's food requirements, and may even reduce their children's risk of developing food allergies in the first place.

Your diet during pregnancy: Although it's controversial, some studies suggest that consumption of high amounts of potentially allergenic foods (such as peanuts or shellfish) by a mother-to-be during pregnancy may trigger allergies in infants. This doesn't mean that expectant mothers should go on a restrictive diet—good nutrition is the cornerstone of a healthy pregnancy. It makes sense, however, that if you have food allergies in the immediate family (a parent, grandparent, or sibling), you avoid gorging on any particular food during pregnancy, especially those most likely to trigger an allergic response in children. Given the fact that peanut allergy is becoming more common, and can be such a serious health threat, I would advise moms-to-be to pass on the peanuts.

Breast feeding: Breast milk is the best milk for babies, period. It's not only the most nutritious, but it helps an infant develop a healthy, well-functioning immune system that could prevent the onset of allergy and asthma. In fact, breast-fed infants have a lower rate of both problems than non-breast-fed. If you have a child with a family history of food allergies, pediatricians recommend breast feeding for at least the first year (and longer if possible), gradually introducing solid foods to your infant, one at a time, so you can determine if there is an allergic reaction. It's best to devise a feeding strategy for your child under the supervision of an informed medical professional who is sensitive to the allergy issue. Although infants are not allergic to their mother's breast milk, they can be allergic to proteins that pass to them via her breast milk. Therefore, during breast feeding, it's advisable for nursing mothers to abstain from foods that other family members may be allergic to. Once again, I think it's smart to avoid peanuts and shellfish, two foods that can trigger potentially life-threatening allergic reactions. Keep track of what you eat. If you see that your child gets colicky or seems in distress after eating a particular food, don't eat it! Eczema (a skin rash) is another sign that your infant may have a food allergy. If breast feeding is not possible, ask your physician about special formulas called hydrolysates, which have a low risk of allergy.

Milk allergy: If your child is allergic to milk, or if your pediatrician suspects that he might be, soy-based formula is another option. However, about 25 percent of all infants who are allergic to dairy will also be allergic to soy. Once again, if your physician is worried that a soy allergy is possible, he or she may prescribe a special low-allergy formula.

Become an educated parent: If you have an allergic child, for the safety of your child, you need to become an authority on food allergies in general, and his or her food allergy in particular. Fortunately, there are some terrific websites run by support groups of parents of allergic children who can provide specific information on the ins and outs of avoiding your child's allergen. In particular, these websites list acceptable products that do not contain allergens and offer alerts on products that may contain allergens that are not stated on the label. (See the Resources section for more information.)

Educate your child's caregivers: It's important for your child's grandparents, baby-sitters, and the parents of his or her friends to understand what food allergy is and why eating certain foods may be harmful to your child. Be sure to keep a list of foods that your child should not eat posted on your refrigerator. Have enough allergy-free foods around so that caregivers can feed your child a snack if he or she gets hungry. If your child spends a great deal of time at a friend's house, ask if you can keep some safe snacks for your child at that house.

Alert teachers and school staff: If your child has a serious allergy—for example, to peanuts—you must alert his or her teacher as well as the school's administrative staff. Most schools are woefully uninformed about allergic children. It's not enough to simply mention the problem to one teacher. Your child may have an allergic reaction outside the classroom, particularly in areas where food is served. It's critical that *all* of your child's caregivers at school, from the cafeteria staff to the school nurse, know what to do in case your child is accidentally exposed to the allergen. Should your child take an antihistamine if he or she shows signs of an allergic reaction? How can you reach his or her doctor? Should your child be taken to an emergency room? Does your child carry an epinephrine injector and when is it appropriate to use it? Who is responsible for storing your child's medication at school? A few minutes of planning can save precious minutes in getting your child the right care, and may even save his or her life. It's a good idea for your child to wear a medic alert tag alerting people to his allergy.

Don't make your child feel deprived: Fortunately, there are numerous allergy-safe products appearing on the shelves in supermarkets and natural food stores. It's possible to find a good-tasting, nondairy, wheat-free, gluten-free cookie or muffin that your child will enjoy. If your child can't eat real ice cream, he or she may be able to eat fruit sorbet or soy-based ice cream, or a "milk" shake made out of rice milk. If your child can't have a birthday cake made out of wheat flour, bake him or her a cake with rice or potato flour. Flourless cakes can be quite delicious. For some excellent flourless cake recipes, check out any kosher cookbook. During the spring Passover holiday, Jews abstain from eating leavened bread, which prohibits the use of products such as yeast and baking powder that make breads and cakes "rise" and give these foods their texture. Ingenious kosher chefs have come up with some wonderful alternatives that do not require flour and would not contain gluten.

There is light at the end of the tunnel: Many children outgrow their food allergies, which is why there are more allergic children than allergic adults. In addition, as your child gets older, he or she will be better able to monitor his or her own food intake and will have a better understanding of the consequences of eating the wrong food, which will take a load off your shoulders.

GENETICALLY MODIFIED FOOD

You are highly allergic to corn, so you are scrupulous about reading food labels to make sure that they do not contain any corn-derived products or additives. In fact, you avoid processed foods and eat lots of fresh vegetables to avoid inadvertently eating corn. But after eating a salad with sliced tomato, you suddenly have an allergy attack, much as you would after eating corn. You wonder, "How could this happen?" You later find out that the tomato has been genetically modified—or altered—to make it more resistant against a certain fungus that targets tomato. Unfortunately, the fungus-resistant gene added to the tomato actually came from a new breed of corn! This hypothetical situation has not happened . . . yet. It is the nightmare scenario presented by opponents of the genetic modification or genetic engineering of the food supply. Genetic modification entails various techniques of altering existing genes within a fruit or vegetable plant or transferring genes from one species to the other to "improve" upon nature's design. For example, if one particular plant species is resistant against a bacteria or an insect pest, or has a high vitamin content, it may be possible to transfer that good trait to a different species of plant. This is nothing new—cross-fertilization of plants to produce desired effects has been practiced for years—however, plant breeders had a limited gene pool to choose from. With the new genetic biotechnology, it's now possible to mix animal DNA with plant DNA, and to produce hybrids that would never occur in nature. For example, in real life, you can't breed a corn plant with a tomato plant any more than you can breed a cat with a dog. In the world of biotech food, however, a tomato plant can be genetically altered to contain genes from a corn plant and still look and smell like a tomato. So, if scientists are creating a better tomato, what's the problem? Proponents argue that there is none, and that genetic engineering will benefit people by producing, among other things, heartier crops that require less pesticide, and even food that is more nutritious than food produced by nature. In fact, supporters point out that much of the fresh produce in the stores today is a result of bioengineering techniques, and that food manufacturers are already using genetically modified plants in their products.

There are several unresolved issues that concern people like myself. For one thing, we don't know the long-term effects of eating genetically altered food. Second, we fear that the next generation of biotech food is going to contain so many weird, unrelated genes that it could make life miserable for allergic people. The question is, when you transfer a gene—or protein—from one unrelated plant species to another, are you also transferring an allergen? Given the fact that some highly allergic people can react to a minuscule amount of allergen, the answer is probably yes, particularly for potent allergenic foods like peanuts or corn. Under proposed new labeling requirements, the FDA will require food manufacturers to alert consumers to the fact that a genetically altered fruit or vegetable may contain a potential allergen. The problem is, the food industry has not done a good job of labeling regular foods. Why should we expect that they will do a better job labeling genetically engineered foods? And what happens when a genetically engineered food, like a tomato, is used to make a packaged tomato sauce? Who is going to track this food to see where it actually turns up?

There are other causes of concern with genetic engineering. It's possible for pollen from genetically modified crops to blow into other areas, possibly even organic farms or the land of farmers trying to raise nonengineered crops. Which raises another question: How will humans react to this new breed of pollen? What about the animals that are exposed to these crops? How will genetic engineering affect insect life—and ultimately, the entire food chain? In one alarming study conducted at Cornell University, monarch butterflies were killed by eating pollen from genetically modified corn that had fallen on their primary food source, milkweed. The corn was engineered to produce a potent herbicide, which was designed to keep it safe from caterpillar predators that destroy corn crops, but had the unintended effect of wiping out nonpest caterpillars that develop into monarch butterflies. Another scary thought—what if this antibug corn actually produces a species of resistant insects that can no longer be controlled by the pesticide in the corn? Due to pressure from consumer groups, many major manufacturers have rejected genetically modified ingredients in their products. At the very least, consumers should have a choice, and food manufacturers should be required to label products using genetically modified foods or additives. The bottom line: More research is needed before we embrace the brave new world of genetically modified food.

FOOD IN UNLIKELY PLACES

Vegetable oils derived from corn, peanuts, or soy are common emollients used in skin lotions, shaving creams, and even lipstick. If you are highly allergic to any of these oils, check with the manufacturer before using any of these products.

CHAPTER 11

Living Well with Asthma

As I write this chapter on asthma on a hot, hazy summer day, I hear on the news that there is an ozone alert throughout most major metropolitan centers of the United States, including LA, where I live. Ozone is released when sunlight hits the fumes emitted by the fuel-burning engines of diesel machinery, trucks, and cars. The newscaster notes that ozone is a serious public health problem and reports that if you have allergies or respiratory problems, ozone may worsen your condition, causing a tightening in the chest, an irritated throat, and a cough, and may even trigger asthma in some people. Her advice: Try to stay indoors until it passes.

Upon hearing this report, I ask myself, is it any wonder that the incidence of asthma has doubled in the United States since the 1980s, leaving 15 million Americans—many of them small children—gasping for air?

Asthma is a chronic inflammatory lung condition. An asthma attack is characterized by a narrowing of the air passages in the lungs, making breathing difficult. About 7 percent of all children are diagnosed with asthma, but as many as twice that many children may have asthmalike symptoms without being diagnosed. You can also develop asthma as an adult, although this is more common in women than in men. Asthma can be mild—so mild that it rarely flares up, and may disappear for years—or it can be serious, and in rare cases, even fatal. Over time, if a severe case goes untreated, it can destroy delicate lung tissue, resulting in even more severe problems, including COPD. Symptoms include coughing, wheezing, and tightness of the chest. The bottom line is, when you have an asthma attack you can't get enough oxygen into your lungs, and ultimately, into your body.

Once rare, asthma has been a growing public health problem since the end of the twentieth century, and it continues to plague us in the twenty-first century. Why the sudden and dramatic increase? Although there is no one answer, the extraordinary increase in pollution, primarily due to automobiles and trucks, is considered a likely cause. Ozone is a particularly potent lung irritant, and one that is difficult to avoid. Allergy—especially if it goes untreated—can also lead to asthma. The increase in exposure to new chemicals and toxins in the environment and food may also be triggers. Genetics is also a factor. A child with one asthmatic parent has a 20 percent chance of developing asthma, a child with two asthmatic parents has a 50 percent chance. But this doesn't explain the increased incidence of asthma in recent years—the fact is, our genetics haven't changed over the past hundred years, so it's not likely that genetics is the primary culprit. More likely, something in the environment, diet, or lifestyle is turning on genes that predispose people to asthma.

Most people with mild cases of asthma learn to manage their illness on their own and rarely seek medical attention. Before I go any further, let me state emphatically that anyone who has serious asthma needs to be treated by a knowledgeable physician. If asthma is interfering with your life, if your symptoms are getting worse, or if you are having frequent asthma attacks and can't control your symptoms, you must get help. The standard drug treatments—inhalers and the like—can help control symptoms and save lives. I am in no way encouraging people to stop taking their medication if they need it. But as a trained pharmacist, I know that drugs have their drawbacks. As a nutritionist and vitamin specialist, I know that it is often possible to control your symptoms by making simple changes in your lifestyle and diet. My goal is to help people reduce their need for powerful medications that can have powerful side effects. To achieve that goal, people must understand how the environment, their diet, and their lifestyle can affect their asthma symptoms. They must be able to identify the particular triggers that can worsen their asthma, making them more and more reliant on medicine. The better educated you are about your problem, the better you will be able to take care of yourself, and the less likely it is you will become overly dependent on drugs.

THE POLLUTION CONNECTION

A recent study of California children by the University of California uncovered a surprising statistic: In communities with the most smog, the most athletic children were *three times* more likely than sedentary children to get asthma. The researchers followed more than thirty-five hundred kids, ages nine to sixteen, with no history of asthma for five years. Out of that group, 8 percent of the kids were doing three or more sports. Children who played their sports in areas with high ozone pollution had significantly higher rates of asthma than kids who did not take part in sports. In other words, the fittest kids were at greater risk of developing asthma! However, kids who played more than three sports did not show a higher incidence of asthma if they lived in low-ozone areas. The researchers hypothesized that the athletic kids living in polluted areas were taking high quantities of ozone into their lungs because during exertion, they take deep, rapid breaths. On the other hand, sedentary kids who sit in front of the TV set or play video games are not exposed to the same amount of ozone.

The study isn't implicating exercise as a cause of asthma, although there is a condition known as exercise-induced asthma that I'll discuss later. The point of this study is that if you live in an ozone-polluted area, you must be aware of pollution levels and ozone alert days. It is foolish to exercise vigorously outdoors on days when the air quality is poor, especially if it only forces you to use more asthma medication, notably inhalers. On days when the air is foul, take your exercise routine indoors, preferably where it is air-conditioned and the air is filtered. Some of you may feel that if you don't get in your daily run or walk, you're endangering your health. The fact is, if you try to work out outdoors in heavy pollution, you are at risk of overtaxing and ultimately harming your lungs.

Of course, if you have the desire and the means, you

can move to an area with no pollution, but changing your habits may be a bit easier than changing your address.

The other step we can take is to support legislation to clean up the air. The governor of California just signed a law that will require cleaner emission standards for automobiles within the next decade. Since California accounts for 10 percent of the automobiles sold in the United States, this could make a real difference in air quality throughout the United States.

EXERCISE-INDUCED ASTHMA

Outdoor exercise, particularly in cold weather, can induce asthma symptoms such as wheezing, shortness of breath, and bronchospasm even in people who may not normally have asthma under other circumstances. Exercise-induced asthma is triggered by the heavier breathing required during exercise, which causes tiny cells in the bronchial tube (bronchioles) to twitch, thereby restricting air flow. If this happens to you, tell your doctor. He or she may suggest that you use an inhaler before you exercise to keep your airways open. Try wearing an outdoor exercise mask around your mouth to warm and moisten the cold, dry outdoor air. These masks will also filter out some pollutants, which is also better for your lungs, and may reduce the need to use your inhalers or "rescue" medication. Once again, exercise common sense. It may be advisable to forgo your run or jog on days when the air is especially dry and cold. If you're not allergic to mold or chlorine, swimming in an indoor pool is great for people with exercise-induced asthma. It's easier on the lungs and is actually good for the bronchial tubes.

CHECK YOUR MEDICINE CABINET

Are you taking any medication that could be aggravating your asthma? Common drug triggers include over-the-counter medicines such as aspirin, nonsteroidal anti-inflammatory drugs such as ibuprofen, and prescription drugs such as ACE inhibitors and beta blockers used to treat heart conditions. Please note that if you are sensitive to aspirin, you may also be sensitive to aspirin substitutes such as acetaminophen. Do be careful when buying over-the-counter cold or allergy medicine—it often includes aspirin or an aspirin substitute. Once again, the best approach is to read the labels carefully. To be on the safe side, before taking any medication, ask your physician or pharmacist if it could worsen your asthma.

ARE YOU EATING AN ASTHMA-PROMOTING DIET?

What you eat has a profound effect on your overall health, and both directly and indirectly affects asthma. In particular, eating a diet laden with refined sugar will worsen both allergy and asthma symptoms, for several reasons. A high-sugar diet can dampen immune function, making you more vulnerable to infection, a common trigger for asthma symptoms. Second, a high-sugar diet promotes inflammation, which will aggravate any existing medical condition, including asthma. Finally, if you're loading up on junk, in all likelihood you're not eating good stuff like fruits and vegetables, which are filled with beneficial antioxidants that reduce inflammation, and prevent free radical damage, which can harm lung tissue.

Foods containing refined sugar also tend to contain lots of food dyes and additives, some of which may also trigger asthma symptoms. Sulfites, used to preserve the color and freshness of food and often added to beer and wine, are a particular problem for asthma sufferers. In addition, a high-sugar diet promotes the growth of candida albicans in the gut, a yeast infection which may exacerbate asthma symptoms in susceptible people.

Are you eating enough good fats, such as omega 3 fatty acids found in fatty freshwater fish and flaxseed? These good fats reduce inflammation and normalize immune function. On the other hand, bad fats, such as transfatty acids found in many processed foods, promote inflammation and the formation of free radicals. In addition to eating foods with good fats, it's a good idea to take an essential fatty acid supplement.

If you have asthma, it's especially important for you to avoid any food allergens that could worsen your symptoms. Please read over the chapter on food allergies: You may have an allergy to a common food and not even know it.

Avoid sugary fruit juices and soda. Instead drink eight to ten glasses of pure, filtered water daily, especially if you are on any medication.

IS STRESS MAKING IT WORSE?

Stress—either good or bad—can make any chronic condition worse, including asthma. Studies have shown that half of all asthma patients feel a constriction in their chest when they're excited—when they're either very happy or very distressed. This is not to suggest that asthma is "all in your head." The fact is, strong emotions can stimulate the autonomic nervous system, which controls such automatic functions as the beating of the heart (you know how your heart starts to race when you're scared or nervous), blood pressure, and breathing. Some researchers believe that just as some people are more likely to get headaches or have stomach troubles when they're upset, there is a group of people who are genetically programmed to develop asthma symptoms when they are upset.

If you're under a great deal of stress, you are more likely to have asthma symptoms. Sadly, asthmatic children who live in homes that are plagued with family conflict and depression are especially vulnerable to extremely severe asthma. It's also true that living with a chronic illness in itself can be very stressful. In fact, relaxation techniques, such breathing exercises, hypnotherapy, and even yoga have proven to be helpful for asthmatics, as I will describe in Chapter 13.

HAVE YOU ALLERGY PROOFED YOUR SURROUNDINGS?

If allergies irritate your asthma, it's worth the investment in time and money to try to allergy proof your home.

Keeping allergens such as dust mites and pollen at bay can go a long way in helping to reduce your symptoms. Avoid exposure to fumes and irritating fragrances in your home. Buy unscented products that are not laden with harsh chemicals. And avoid inhaling cigarette smoke—yours or somebody else's. Tobacco smoke is a common asthma trigger.

If you are irritated by chemicals in the workplace, work with your employer to reduce your exposure. Review Chapter 7 to see what you can do to make your workplace work for you.

CHAPTER 12

A Guide to Antiallergy Drugs

BY PRESCRIPTION ONLY

It seems that every year, a new antiallergy drug is brought to market with a great deal of fanfare, including full-page ads in popular magazines and prime-time television commercials. The cost of promotion is built into the hefty price tag—no wonder prescription drug prices are skyrocketing! Each new drug promises to be better than the old drugs, but the reality is, most antiallergy drugs are pretty similar. In all fairness, on occasion, there is a true pharmaceutical breakthrough in the treatment of allergy. (The newer, nonsedating antihistamines that I discuss below are a prime example.) In many cases, however, allergy has become such a "growth industry" that every pharmaceutical house wants to have its entry in this lucrative market whether or not it has anything new to offer. Before you get seduced by the pricey new kid on the block, you should know what antiallergy drugs really are, and how they work.

Antihistamines, the primary class of drugs used to treat allergies, inhibit the action of histamine, the chemical that is produced by mast cells after exposure to an allergen. Histamine works by attaching itself to special sites on cells called receptors. Think of the receptor as a lock and histamine as the key. Histamine "unlocks" the receptor to begin the allergic cascade that causes allergic symptoms. Antihistamines attach themselves to the same receptors on cells as histamine, which prevents histamine from binding to these sites, thus dampening the allergic response. The older antihistamines (Benadryl, Atarax, Tavist, Dimetapp, and so forth), which are sold over the counter, work well but cause drowsiness. The newer, more expensive nonsedating antihistamines (Claritin, Clarinex, Allegra, and Zyrtec) are available only by prescription, with the exception of Claritin. Antihistamines are used both to prevent and to treat allergic reactions, but the earlier you catch an allergy, the more effective the antihistamine. That's why people are advised to begin their seasonal antiallergy therapy a month or two before symptoms set in. Antihistamines don't always work because they only target histamine and are not effective against other allergic mediators, including leukotrienes and other inflammatory cells. In some cases, antihistamines may dampen an allergic response, but not stop it. In addition, the effect of an antihistamine is short-lived; you need to take it every day to control allergy. If you take the same antihistamine for a long period of time, it could become ineffective against your symptoms, which means that you will have to switch to a different drug. If allergy is a trigger for their asthma, asthmatics may also take antihistamines along with antiasthmatic medication. However, antihistamines alone are not used to treat asthma.

There are two types of drugs prescribed for asthma: anti-inflammatory medicines and bronchodilators. Anti-inflammatory medicines target specific immune cells such as leukotrienes, which promote inflammation and damage the lungs. Bronchodilators are muscle relaxers that relieve bronchial spasm and open up the airways to allow normal breathing. Some bronchodilators are short-acting and are to be used solely as rescue medication to stop an asthma attack. Others are long-acting—they work to prevent an asthma attack but may not be useful to stop one. The short-acting drugs are powerful drugs that can have significant side effects, and are to be used only as directed by your doctor. The problem with bronchodilators is that they may restore breathing but mask the underlying inflammation. When it comes to asthma, it's very important to take a holistic approach and try to control the triggers in your life that can aggravate the condition, whether that trigger is pollution, stress, an infection, or an indoor or outdoor allergy. Don't wait until you're gasping for breath!

Cromoglycate type drugs (known by the generic name cromolyn) are used only to prevent allergic reactions—once an allergy hits, they are of little use. Cromolyn is a mast cell stabilizer—that is, it blocks the allergic response early in the game, long before the mast cells release histamine. These drugs are a more sophisticated version of the old-fashioned antihistamines, but don't work as well as antihistamines to stop an allergic reaction after the fact.

Antihistamine alone or antihistamine and mast cell stabilizer combinations are used in ophthalmic solutions to treat itchy, allergic eyes.

Steroid nasal sprays are typically prescribed for asthma and allergy. Steroids are similar to the corticosteroids produced by the adrenal glands. They are potent anti-inflammatories and are not to be taken casually. Steroid inhalers are used for asthma. Low-dose steroid inhalers are considered relatively safe as compared to oral steroids.

Steroid pills may be prescribed for cases of severe allergy or asthma. Short-term use (no more than three weeks) of these drugs is considered safe, but long-term use can cause severe problems, including increased susceptibility to infection, puffiness, thinning of the bones, diabetes, high blood pressure, and mood changes. Steroid pills must be tapered off slowly, or you can cause severe rebound problems. If you are becoming overly reliant on steroids, it's a sign that you need to reassess your lifestyle and better understand the activities or stresses in your life that trigger severe asthma or allergic reactions.

Depending on the severity of the problem, the treatment of asthma is complicated and varies from patient to patient. Don't discontinue taking your medicine, or change your medicine, except under the supervision of your physician. I've said it before but it's worth repeating here. My goal is to enable you to live a healthy life, as drug-free as possible, but I can't guarantee that you will never need medicine. If you have a severe asthma or allergy attack, it's good to know that there is reliable "rescue" medication available.

People often ask me if there are any advantages to prescription drugs versus over-the-counter drugs. My answer is, it depends on several factors, ranging from your particular health needs to your pocketbook. In some cases, you may not have a choice. There may not be an over-the-counter alternative to the drug you need, particularly if you are using one of the new asthma drugs that I describe below. These drugs require the close supervision of a medical expert, and I doubt that they will ever be sold over the counter. Until very recently, you could not buy a nonsedating antihistamine without a prescription. As of this writing, Claritin is being introduced as an over-the-counter drug, and my hunch is, other manufacturers will be bringing out their versions of this drug soon.

Still, even if you have an over-the-counter option, it may make economic sense for you to use a prescription drug if it is covered by insurance, since over-the-counter drugs usually are not. Of course, prescription drugs are a lot more expensive, and if you pay a hefty deductible on every prescription (some people pay twenty dollars or more), it could still be cheaper to buy an over-the-counter antihistamine for just a few dollars. If you are forced to use a prescription drug, please keep in mind that generic brands are just as good as brand names, and are usually a fraction of the cost. Ask your doctor to prescribe a generic brand if possible.

In the section below, I review the top prescription drugs for asthma and allergy. I also list the primary side effects associated with each drug. If you are taking any of these drugs, it doesn't mean that you will have any side effects, but I want you to be aware that it's possible.

Natural Antihistamines

Natural antihistamines include Tylophora, butterbur, vitamin C, Chinese skullcap, green tea, perilla, and reishi (see Hot 55 Antiallergy Supplements).

Top Prescription Drugs

Brand name: ACCOLATE (tablets)
Generic name: Zafirlukast
Drug type: Leukotriene inhibitor (anti-inflammatory) that inhibits bronchoconstriction, opening up the airways
Use: For the treatment of chronic asthma
Principal side effects: Headache, infection, nausea, diarrhea, generalized pain, weakness, abdominal pain, accidental injury, dizziness, myalgia, fever, back pain, vomiting, and upset stomach

Brand name: ADVAIR DISKUS (inhaler)
Generic name: Fluticasone propionate
Drug type: Synthetic steroidal anti-inflammatory
Use: For the long-term, twice-daily maintenance treatment of asthma in people twelve years of age and older
Principal side effects: Gastrointestinal discomfort and pain, musculoskeletal pain, upper respiratory infection, pharyngitis, upper respiratory inflammation, sinusitis, hoarseness, dysphonia (altered voice production), oral yeast (fungal) infection, viral respiratory infection, bronchitis, cough, headache, nausea, vomiting, and diarrhea

Brand name: AEROBID INHALER (inhaler by mouth)
Generic name: Flunisolide
Drug type: Synthetic steroidal anti-inflammatory
Use: This inhaler is indicated in the maintenance

treatment of asthma as a prophylactic therapy. On a positive note, patients who require systemic steroids (taken orally) may find that Aerobid may reduce their need for steroids. This inhaler is not indicated for the relief of acute bronchospasm.

Principal side effects: Diarrhea, nausea and vomiting, upset stomach, sore throat, headache, cold symptoms, nasal congestion, upper respiratory infection, unpleasant taste, palpitations, abdominal pain, heartburn, chest pain, yeast infection, dizziness, irritability, nervousness, shakiness, decreased appetite, swelling, fever, menstrual distress, chest congestion, cough, hoarseness, rhinitis, runny nose, sinus congestion, sinus drainage, sinus infection, sinusitis, wheezing, pharyngitis, phlegm and throat irritation, anxiety, depression, faintness, vertigo, hyperactivity, hypoactivity, insomnia, moodiness, numbness, chills, increased appetite and weight gain, malaise, peripheral edema, sweating, weakness, hypertension, rapid heartbeat, constipation, upset stomach, gas, bruising, enlarged lymph nodes, dry throat, inflammation of the tongue, mouth irritation, eye discomfort, eye infection, bronchitis, chest tightness, dyspnea, nosebleeds, head stuffiness, nasal irritation, pleurisy, pneumonia, sinus discomfort, acne, hives, urticaria, blurred vision, and fatigue

Brand name: AEROLATE SR., AEROLATE JR., THEO-DUR (tablet, capsule, or liquid)
Generic name: Theophylline
Drug type: Caffeine-type drug that relieves bronchospasm

Use: A bronchodilator used for the treatment of chronic asthma and other chronic lung diseases, this drug is most often combined with another prescription drug, Rynatuss.

Principal side effects: Nausea, vomiting, epigastric pain, palpitations, headache, and dizziness

Brand name: ALLEGRA AND ALLEGRA-D (capsules and tablets)

Generic name: Fexofenadine HCL and fexofenadine and pseudoephedrine HCL-A decongestant

Drug type: Nonsedating oral antihistamine

Use: Seasonal allergy and allergy related hives—Allegra and Allegra-D (the D is for decongestant) are the new variety of nonsedating antihistamines. Although not listed as a primary side effect, some people find that if they take Allegra-D too close to bedtime, it can interfere with sleep.

Principal side effects for twelve years and older: Susceptibility to colds, flu, nausea, menstrual problems, drowsiness, dyspepsia, fatigue, headache, upper respiratory infections, back pain

Principal side effects for younger than twelve years: Headache, accidental injury, coughing, fever, pain, earache, upper respiratory infections

Brand name: ATROVENT (inhaler and nasal spray)

Generic name: Ipratroprium bromide

Drug type: Bronchodilator—anticholerginic agent, relaxes muscles by blocking the action of the parasympathetic or "involuntary" nervous system

Use: For the treatment of bronchospasm associated

with COPD, emphysema, and maintenance treatment of chronic bronchitis

Principal side effects: Nosebleeds, pharyngitis, upper respiratory infection, nasal dryness, headache, dry mouth, dry throat, difficulty tasting food, sinusitis, pain, and diarrhea

Brand name: AZMACORT (inhalation aerosol)
Generic name: Triamcinolone acetonide
Drug type: Synthetic steroidal anti-inflammatory
Use: For the treatment of seasonal allergies and perennial allergic inflammation of the nasal mucous membranes
Principal side effects: Sinusitis, pharyngitis, headache, facial swelling, pain, abdominal pain, photosensitivity, weight gain, bursitis, myalgia, cystitis, urinary tract infections, diarrhea, toothache, vomiting, dry mouth, oral yeast infections, rash, chest congestion, voice alteration, and vaginal yeast infection

Brand name: BECONASE (inhalation aerosol)
Generic name: Beclomethasone dipropionate
Drug type: Synthetic steroidal anti-inflammatory nasal spray
Use: Relief of symptoms of seasonal or perennial allergic and nonallergic rhinitis
Principal side effects: Sensations of irritation and burning in the nose, sneezing attacks, unpleasant taste and smell, loss of taste and smell, rhinorrhea, yeast infections of the nose and pharynx, nosebleeds,

headaches, lightheadedness, dryness and irritation of the nose and throat

Brand name: BECONASE AQ and VANCERIL INHALER
Generic name: Beclomethasone dipropionate
Drug type: Synthetic steroidal anti-inflammatory
Use: For the relief of the symptoms of seasonal or perennial allergic and nonallergic rhinitis
Principal side effects: Irritation of the nasal mucous membranes, urticaria, rash, bronchospasm, sneezing attacks, headache, nausea and lightheadedness, nasal stuffiness, nosebleeds, rhinorrhea, tearing eyes, dryness and irritation of the nose and throat, unpleasant taste and smell, loss of taste and smell, and wheezing

Brand Name: CLARINEX (tablets and syrup)
Generic Name: Desloratadine
Drug type: Nonsedating oral antihistamine
Use: Seasonal allergy and perennial allergy. Although Clarinex is being promoted as the new kid on the block, it is basically the same drug as Claritin (loratadine), an antihistamine that typically does not induce drowsiness in most people. Claritin is assimilated in the body as desloratadine, hence the "new" drug. Why the change? Claritin's patent is running out, and this slightly altered formulation gives the pharmaceutical company a new twenty-year patent. The original Claritin is now sold over the counter without a prescription and has always been available in Canada without a prescription. Since most insur-

ance companies in the United States will not reimburse for a nonprescription drug, it's critical for a drug company to offer a prescription drug or risk losing market share.

Principal side effects: Inflammation of the pharynx (the upper extended portion of the digestive tube), dry mouth, headache, myalgia (muscle pain), nausea, fatigue, dizziness, sleepiness, upset stomach, dysmenorrhea (difficult or painful menstruation), tachycardia (rapid heartbeat)

Brand name: COMBIVENT (inhaler)

Generic name: Ipratropium bromide and albuterol sulfate

Drug type: Anticholinergic bronchodilator and Beta 2-adrenergic bronchodilator. It works by relaxing the smooth muscle tissue to relieve bronchospasm and open up the airways.

Use: For the secondary treatment of Chronic Obstructive Pulmonary Disease (COPD), Combivent is indicated for people with COPD on a regular aerosol bronchodilator who continue to have bronchospasm and who require a secondary bronchodilator.

Principal side effects: Headache, pain, flu, chest pain, nausea, bronchitis, dyspnea, cough, respiratory disorders, pneumonia, bronchospasm, upper respiratory infection, pharyngitis, sinusitis, and inflammation of the nasal mucous membrane

Brand name: FLONASE (nasal spray)

Generic name: Fluticasone propionate

Drug type: Synthetic steroidal anti-inflammatory

Use: Fluticasone is a steroid produced by the adrenal glands. Flonase is used to treat nasal symptoms of seasonal allergies and chronic inflammation of the nasal mucous membrane for adults and children four years of age and older. It may be used in combination with oral antihistamines.

Principal side effects: Headache, pharyngitis (inflammation of the pharynx), nosebleeds, cough, nasal burning and irritation, nausea, vomiting, and asthma symptoms

Brand name: FLOVENT (oral inhaler)

Generic name: Fluticasone propionate

Drug type: Synthetic steroidal anti-inflammatory

Use: Similar to Flonase, this drug is for the maintenance treatment of asthma as prophylactic therapy for adults and children four years of age and older. If you use this drug, you have to be vigilant about rinsing your mouth out with water after each use, or risk getting an oral yeast infection.

Principal side effects: Upper respiratory infections, throat irritations, sinusitis, upper respiratory inflammation, inflammation of nasal mucous membrane, oral yeast (fungus), nausea, vomiting, stomach distress, fever, viral infection, cough, bronchitis, headache, muscle injury, musculoskeletal pain, injury

Brand name: MAXAIR INHALER

Generic name: Pirbuterol acetate

Drug Type: Bronchodilator—short-acting Beta-2 reliever, mimics the role of epinephrine in the body

Use: For the prevention and reversal of bronchospasm in people twelve years or older, it may be used with or without concurrent theophylline or steroid therapy.

Principal side effects: Tremors, nervousness, headaches, weakness, drowsiness, dizziness, palpitations, rapid heartbeat, chest pain, tightness, cough, nausea, diarrhea, dry mouth, vomiting, skin reaction, rash, bruising, smell and taste change, backache, fatigue, hoarseness, and nasal congestion

Brand Name: NASACORT (nasal spray and solution)
Generic name: Triamcinolone acetonide
Drug type: Steroidal anti-inflammatory
Use: For the treatment of the nasal symptoms of seasonal and perennial allergy in adults and children age six and over
Principal side effects: Nosebleeds, cough, fever, nausea, throat discomfort, inflammation of the ear, stomach upset

Brand name: NASALCROM, INTAL, GASTRO-CROM, CROLOM (ophthalmic solution)
Generic name: Cromolyn sodium USP 24
Drug Type: Antihistamine–mast cell inhibitor
Use: Preventive only for allergy and asthma. Cromolyn sodium 4 percent ophthalmic solution is used to treat allergic eyes.
Principal side effects: Headache, diarrhea, nausea, myalgia, abdominal pain, rash, and irritability

Brand name: NASONEX (nasal spray)

Generic name: Mometasone furoate monohydrate
Drug type: Synthetic steroidal anti-inflammatory
Use: Treatment of the nasal symptoms of seasonal allergic and perennial allergic rhinitis in adults and children three years and older
Principal side effects: Headache, viral infection, pharyngitis (inflammation of the pharynx), blood-tinged mucus, cough, upper respiratory infection, dysmenorrhea, musculoskeletal pain, sinusitis, vomiting

Brand name: PATANOL (ophthalmic solution)
Generic name: Olopatadine hydrochloride
Drug type: Antihistamine, mast cell inhibitor
Use: The leading prescription drug for the treatment of allergic conjunctivitis
Principal side effects: Headaches, asthma, blurred vision, burning or stinging of the eyes, cold syndrome, allergic rhinitis, foreign body sensation, keratitis, lid edema, nausea, pharyngitis, pruritus, hyperemia, general allergic symptoms (could be from underlying allergy), dry eye, taste perversion

Brand name: PROVENTIL (inhalation solution, inhalation aerosol, and time-released tablets)
Generic name: Albuterol sulfate
Drug type: Bronchodilator—short-acting Beta-2 reliever, similar in action to ephinephrine in the body
Use: For the treatment of bronchospasm for asthmatics twelve years and older. The inhalation aerosol is used for bronchodilation prevention and relief, and the prevention of exercise-related bronchospasm.

The solution inhalation is recommended for relief of bronchospasm for people twelve years of age and older with reversible, obstructed airway disease and acute attacks of bronchospasm.

Principal side effects: Nervousness, headache, dizziness, weakness, sleeplessness, irritability, drowsiness, restlessness, palpitations, rapid heartbeat, flushing, chest discomfort, muscle cramps, nausea, and difficulty urinating

Brand name: RHINOCORT (nasal spray and intranasal inhaler)
Generic name: Budesonide
Drug type: Steroidal anti-inflammatory
Use: For the management of symptoms of seasonal allergies in adults and children and nonallergic rhinitis in adults, Rhinocort is not recommended for the treatment of nonallergic rhinitis in children.
Principal side effects: Nosebleeds, pharyngitis, bronchospasm, coughing, and nasal irritation

Brand name: RYNATUSS (tablet, capsule, or liquid)
Generic name: Ephedrine
Drug type: Antihistamine
Use: Bronchial dilator for chronic asthma and other lung diseases, and nasal decongestant
Principal side effects: Drowsiness, sedation, dryness of mucous membranes, and gastrointestinal distress

Brand name: SEREVENT (inhaler)
Generic name: Salmeterol xinafoate
Drug type: Bronchodilator

Use: Long-acting Beta-2 reliever, Serevent mimics the role of epinephrine in the body. It opens up restricted airways for asthma patients and people with Chronic Obstructive Pulmonary Disease (COPD).

Principal side effects for asthmatics: Upper respiratory infection, nasopharyngitis, sinus headache, stomachache, headache, tremor, cough

Principal side effects for COPD: Upper respiratory infection, diarrhea, sore throat, nasal sinus infection, back pain, headache, and chest congestion

Brand name: SINGULAIR (tablets and chewable tablets)

Generic name: Montelukast sodium

Drug type: Antileukotriene anti-inflammatory—targets immune cells that trigger inflammation and bronchospasm

Use: For prevention and chronic treatment of asthma in adults and children two years of age and older

Principal side effects: Fatigue, fever, abdominal pain, trauma, dizziness, headache, stomach upset, dental pain, stuffy nose, nasal congestion, cough, flu, and rash

Brand name: TUSSIONEX PENNKINETIC EXTENDED-RELEASE SUSPENSION (cough syrup)

Generic name: Hydrocodone polistirex and chlorpheniramine polistirex

Drug type: Narcotic cough suppressant and antihistamine

Principal side effects: Sedation, drowsiness, mental

clouding, anxiety, fear, euphoria, dizziness, psychological dependence, mood changes, rash, itchy skin, nausea, vomiting, constipation, urinary retention, respiratory depression, dryness of the pharynx, and tightness of the chest. Physical dependence and tolerance may occur.

Brand name: ZADITOR OPHTHALMIC SOLUTION
Generic name: Ketofifen fumarate
Drug type: Mast cell stabilizer similar to cromoglycate
Use: Temporary prevention of itching of the eye due to allergic conjunctivitis
Principal side effects: Headaches, rhinitis, burning and stinging in the eye, discharge, keratitis, dry eye, eyelid disorder, photophobia, rash, flu syndrome, pharyngitis

Brand name: ZYRTEC (tablets and syrup)
Generic name: Cetirizine hydrochloride
Drug type: Nonsedating oral antihistamine
Use: Seasonal allergy due to allergens such as ragweed and pollen, and indoor allergies such as dust mites and animal dander for adults and children two years of age and older. Ads for Zyrtec make a big deal about it being the only antihistamine approved by the FDA for both indoor and outdoor allergies. It may be a clever selling point in a market crowded with antiallergy drugs, but the fact is, all antihistamines work pretty much the same way and should be effective against all allergens.

Principal side effects for twelve years and older: Fatigue, sleepiness, dry mouth, pharyngitis (inflammation of the pharynx), and dizziness

Principal side effects for younger than twelve years: Headache, fatigue, pharyngitis (inflammation of the pharynx), abdominal pain, coughing, sleepiness, diarrhea, nosebleed, bronchospasm, nausea, vomiting, dry mouth, and dizziness.

OVER-THE-COUNTER ALLERGY AND SINUS DRUGS

I am always astonished by the number and variety of allergy and cold medicines that are sold over the counter. There are literally scores of products on the shelves, each varying slightly from the others, but if you read ingredient labels carefully, you will see that most of these products contain one or more of the ten ingredients listed below. All contain an antihistamine, but some may also include a painkiller such as acetaminophen or ibuprofen, and others may also have a decongestant. I'm frequently asked which antihistamine is best, but as far as I'm concerned, there is very little difference between antihistamines. Some may work better for some people than others, but the real issue is whether you need to take the nonsedating variety. If you use antihistamines occasionally, and only at night when you can sleep, the older and less expensive antihistamines are fine. If, however, you take antihistamines daily and need to be alert and functioning, you should only use the nonsedating variety. In fact, it can be dangerous to drive or operate heavy machinery if you are taking antihistamines or any drug that can make you drowsy.

If you have a headache or body ache along with your allergy symptoms, you may select a product with a pain reliever. If you have a stuffy nose, you may select a product with a decongestant. Keep in mind, however, that the more drugs you take, the more likely you are to suffer from one or more of the negative side effects listed below. I don't use these drugs, but since so many people do, I think it's important that you understand the risks as well as the benefits. I am frequently asked whether the less expensive store brands or generic brands are as good as the heavily advertised and more expensive brand names. My answer is an emphatic YES! Store brands are just as good as brand names, and kinder to your pocketbook.

Generic name: Acetaminophen

Brand names: Included in all Tylenol products (Tylenol Cold, Tylenol Sinus, Tylenol Severe Allergy, Children's Tylenol Allergy-D, Pyrexate caplets, Triaminic Allergy Soft Chews (pediatric)

Use: Pain reliever; works well for headache and body ache; aspirin free

Principal side effects: Liver damage (do not drink alcohol with this drug, as it can lead to severe liver damage), nervousness, dizziness, sleeplessness

Generic name: Brompheniramine

Brand names: Dimetapp cold/allergy elixir, Robitussin allergy and cold

Use: Antihistamine

Principal side effects: Nervousness, dizziness, sleep-lessness

Generic name: Chlorpheniramine maleate
Brand names: Chlor-Trimeton Allergy, Tylenol Allergy and Sinus
Use: Antihistamine
Principal side effects: Drowsiness, nervousness, sleeplessness

Generic name: Clemastine fumarate
Brand name: Tavist
Use: Antihistamine
Principal side effects: Drowsiness, excitability (especially in children), nervousness, dizziness, sleep-lessness

Generic name: Dexbrompheniramine
Brand names: Drixoral cold and allergy
Use: Anticough
Principal side effects: Nervousness, dizziness, sleep-lessness

Generic name: Diphenhydramine
Brand names: Benadryl tablets, capsules, and liquid, Children's Benadryl allergy liquid, Pyrexate caplets
Use: Antihistamine
Principal side effects: Marked drowsiness, dizziness, nervousness

Generic name: Doxylamine
Brand name: Tylenol sinus

Use: Antihistamine
Principal side effects: Nervousness, dizziness, heart
   palpitations

Generic name: Ibuprofen
Brand names: Advil cold and sinus, Motrin sinus/
   headache
Use: Pain reliever
Principal side effects: Nervousness, dizziness, sleep-
   lessness, stomach pain

Generic name: Naproxen
Brand name: Aleve cold and sinus
Use: Pain reliever
Principal side effects: Allergic reaction, hives, facial
   swelling, wheezing, and shock, pill feels as if it is
   stuck in your throat, heartburn, stomach pain

Generic name: Pseudoephedrine
Brand names: Advil cold and sinus, Tylenol sinus,
   Children's Tylenol Allergy-D, Aleve cold and sinus,
   Motrin sinus/headache, Triaminic Allergy soft chews
   (pediatric), Pyrexate caplets, Tavist sinus, Robitussin
   allergy and cough, Triaminic allergy/congestion pe-
   diatric liquid, Dimetapp cold and allergy elixir,
   Drixoral cold and allergy, Actifed Allergy and Cold
Use: Decongestant
Principal side effects: Nervousness, dizziness, heart
   palpitations

CHAPTER 13

Alternative Treatment Options

Acupuncture to Breathing Therapy to Yoga

ALTERNATIVE MEDICINE—THERAPIES THAT DEPART FROM the standard pharmaceutical model—is growing in popularity in the United States, particularly for chronic medical problems such as allergy and asthma. People are turning to alternative therapies for several reasons. First and foremost, they are looking for ways to reduce symptoms, feel better, and reduce their need for medication. Second, many are not content merely to turn their medical treatment over to their physicians, or to put their trust entirely in pills and inhalers. They are seeking ways to retake control of their lives and achieve a better quality of life.

In the pages that follow, I describe some of the most common forms of alternative medicine that are being used by people with asthma and allergy. If you are interested in pursuing any of them, I urge you to work with a qualified medical practitioner, and I tell you where you can find one. Please do not discontinue any medical treatment on your own, particularly if you have severe allergy or asthma.

The best approach is to form a partnership with your physician or healer, and work together.

ACUPUNCTURE

Acupuncture is part of the traditional Chinese medicine system of diagnosis and treatment that dates back thousands of years. An acupuncture practitioner uses thin, wire needles or finger pressure to stimulate certain points (acupoints) in the body. Western researchers have shown that acupuncture treatment can produce real and measurable physiological changes, including altering the secretion of hormones and neurotransmitters that control pain and mood and help regulate organ systems. In fact, in the West, acupuncture is used for specific medical purposes, such as treating back pain, arthritis, or headaches. But Chinese practitioners of acupuncture do not regard acupuncture as a treatment for specific conditions. Instead, it is used to correct the body's vital energy, which they call "chi." Unlike medical practitioners in the West, where each malady is believed to be caused by a specific medical problem, TCM practitioners believe that all illness is a result of a disruption in energy flow in one or more systems of the body, which can be corrected through acupuncture. They divide the body into different acupuncture points, each controlling the energy flow to a different organ or system. Although these concepts are foreign to the West, acupuncture has gained popularity in recent years, particularly for the treatment of chronic ailments that cannot be cured by Western drugs, including asthma and allergy.

There have been several studies documenting the benefits of acupuncture treatment for allergy and asthma, but they have their limitations, at least in terms of Western medicine. Due to the nature of acupuncture, it's difficult to design placebo-controlled double-blind studies, the gold standard for Western scientists. In a placebo-controlled, double-blind study, there are two groups of subjects, one given the real treatment, and one given a placebo that appears absolutely real. Neither the subjects nor the researchers know who is getting the real treatment and who is getting the placebo. In order to meet these Western standards, a study of acupuncture would have to have a control group receiving some kind of treatment that was similar to acupuncture, but a worthless, sham procedure—that way, both groups would *think* that they were having real acupuncture done, but only one group would actually have had it. It would, of course, be impossible for the people doing the acupuncture not to know which group was getting the real procedure, as opposed to the sham procedure—so there goes your double-blind study. That's why most studies of acupuncture merely track two groups—those who receive the treatment and those who did not—and Western physicians are somewhat skeptical of this research because they feel that it does not factor in the placebo effect.

The studies that have investigated the effectiveness of acupuncture for asthma and allergy have, by and large, yielded positive results. In most studies, patients report significant symptom relief for both allergy and asthma, and a reduction in the need for medicine. Several studies have reported that acupuncture desensitizes the nasal passage to the production of histamine, resulting in less itching. Following acupuncture therapy, researchers have found a significant drop in IgE, the antibody produced by the immune system that triggers allergic symptoms. Depending on the severity of your problem, treatment can entail several visits to the acupuncturist over a period of weeks or even months. If you want to try an acupuncturist, I recommend that you find one who is knowledgeable in allergy and asthma, preferably one with an M.D. To find a skilled acupuncture therapist in your area, contact the American Academy of Medical Acupuncture (AAMA) at www.medicalacupuncture.org.

BREATHING THERAPY

Breathing is an activity that is supposed to come naturally—in fact, we don't even have to think about breathing, we just do it. Like the beating of our hearts, breathing is under the control of the autonomic or involuntary nervous system. But in the middle of the twentieth century, a Russian scientist asked an intriguing question. What if some people are not breathing correctly? And what if abnormal breathing patterns were the true cause of asthma? In the 1940s, Russian physiologist Konstantin Pavolovich Buteyko began investigating the possibility that hyperventilation—breathing too deeply—was the underlying cause of numerous chronic health problems, including asthma, high blood pressure, and anxiety disorders. Buteyko observed that hyperventilation produced many of the symptoms associated with asthma, such as tightness in the chest, especially after exercise, wheezing, breathlessness, and lightheadedness. Hyperventilation can be very uncomfortable, and can make you feel jittery and on edge, but why would it be unhealthy? Buteyko believed that hyperventilation was creating an imbalance between the two key gases that help run the body—oxygen and carbon dioxide. Simply put, when you inhale you take in oxygen, and when you exhale, you give off carbon dioxide. And although we tend to think of oxygen as essential for life, and carbon dioxide as a waste product, in reality, our bodies need to achieve the right balance of both gases to run normally. In particular, carbon dioxide helps maintain the normal acid balance in the body. If you continually hyperventilate, the theory is, you would be altering your body chemistry, causing damage to important body systems, including your heart and lungs.

Buteyko developed the Buteyko Breathing Technique (BBT) that retrains the body to adopt a more shallow breathing pattern that prevents the exhalation of excess carbon dioxide. The BBT technique has a large following in Europe, and is now being taught in the United States. Needless to say, BBT is controversial, primarily because asthma patients following the technique did not show any improvement of their medical symptoms based on objective criteria such as improved pulmonary function. Several studies conducted in Europe, however, have shown that BBT can help asthma patients reduce their need for bronchodilators, and patients typically report an improved quality of life. Is it another example of the power of the placebo? Who knows! To add fuel to the controversy, a recent study appearing in the prestigious British medical journal *The Lancet* reported that based on a self-assessment questionnaire of asthma patients, one third of all women and one fifth of all men had scores that suggested that they had abnormal breathing patterns that could be aggravating, if not causing, their condition. But an editorial in the same journal noted that there was no solid scientific evidence backing the claim that breathing therapy could help asthmatics.

If you're interested in learning more about BBT, contact Buteyko Asthma Education USA, 2507 Brewster Rd., Indianapolis, IN 46268, or call 1-877-278-4623. The group offers BBT instructional videos as well as lists of teachers in your area. Or check out their website, www.buteyko-usa.com.

If you're interested in trying BBT, please work with your physician or natural healer for the best results.

HOMEOPATHY

If you ever wandered through the homeopathic section at your natural food store or pharmacy, you undoubtedly saw row upon row of products with odd-sounding names, such as *Allium cepa* or *Nux vomica,* and strange labels that say things like "6-X" or "200-C," and you may have wondered what it was all about. Although homeopathic products sometimes use herbs, homeopathy is not merely another form of herbal medicine. It is a distinct medical practice founded about two hundred years ago by Samuel Hahnemann, a German physician who rebelled against the then-dangerous practices typical of the medical profession, such as bloodletting and the routine use of highly toxic medicines such as mercury-based laxatives. Dr. Hahnemann had been intrigued by a saying of Hippocrates, "Look for the cure in the cause." From that phrase, Dr.

Hahnemann deduced that the symptoms of disease were actually the body's way of healing itself, and that in order to cure a health problem, the worst thing you could do would be to smother the symptoms. Rather, you needed to bring the symptoms on safely and quickly, so that the body could heal itself. For example, Dr. Hahnemann knew that cinchona bark was a time-honored folk remedy for malaria. As part of his research, he took high doses of cinchona bark and found that he developed high fever and other malaria-type symptoms. When he stopped taking the bark, the symptoms disappeared. Dr. Hahnemann reasoned that if high doses of cinchona caused malarialike symptoms in healthy people, very low doses of cinchona could help bring about a cure in people who had malaria. From this experiment, and numerous others using different remedies, Dr. Hahnemann developed the foundation of homeopathy, which is known as the "Law of Similars," or more simply put, "like cures like." For example, under the Law of Similars, a homeopathic preparation for allergy would not be an antihistamine that blocks allergic symptoms, but pollen or another plant part that, in high doses, would actually aggravate the symptoms. In very low homeopathic doses, however, it could cure the problem. At first glance, this may sound outlandish, but if you think about it, "like cures like" is the underlying science behind vaccination—that is, a tiny amount of a virus can stimulate the body to produce antibodies against a particular disease. It is also similar to immunotherapy—allergy shots—in which small amounts of the allergen are introduced into the body to desensitize the immune system. In both cases, "like cures like," albeit for different reasons.

Dr. Hahnemann spent years researching various remedies and published his findings in his groundbreaking book, *Chronic Diseases: Their Nature and Homeopathic Cure*, which revolutionized the practice of medicine. Dr. Hahnemann not only created a homeopathic pharmacy, but offered advice on which homeopathic preparation worked best for specific personality types. For example, if you were depressed but had a runny nose, you would take a different preparation than if you were irritable and had the same symptoms. In the nineteenth century, homeopathy was a very popular form of medicine, practiced by homeopathic healers and even some physicians. At the beginning of the twentieth century, the American Medical Association was established primarily to run homeopaths out of business because they were taking so much business away from M.D.s! The AMA succeeded, and homeopathy lost its foothold in the United States. In Europe, however, it remains to date a popular form of medicine practiced by many physicians. In recent years, there has been a resurgence in interest in homeopathy in the United States, but it still remains somewhat mysterious and poorly understood.

For one thing, homeopathy defies everything we believe is true in chemistry. According to the rules of homeopathy established by Dr. Hahnemann, the smaller the amount of the active ingredient in the preparation, the more potent the product! In other words, less is more, and a lot less is a lot more. All homeopathic preparations are extremely diluted. A barely traceable amount of active ingredient is mixed in the suspension fluid, so, for example, a product identified as 6-X has been diluted six times, a product labeled 10-X has been diluted ten times. If a substance has been diluted one hundred times, it is described as 1-C. After it is diluted, it goes through another process known as percussing in which it is shaken and tapped. Although at one time this was done by hand, today it is done by machine. Sometimes a homeopathic preparation is rendered so dilute that there is no traceable ingredient left! Yet homeopaths would consider this to be the most potent product of all. This drives scientists crazy because there is no rational reason why homeopathic preparations should work, and yet, many clinical studies have found them to be effective against numerous ailments, from childhood dysentery to rheumatoid arthritis, and yes, even allergy.

Several studies have confirmed that homeopathic preparations can help relieve allergic symptoms, particularly for hay fever. In one famous 1986 study published in the British medical journal *The Lancet*, 150 hay fever patients were given either a homeopathic remedy consisting of a very dilute mixture of pollen or a placebo. Two weeks later, the researchers concluded that those taking the homeopathic remedy had "shown a significant reduction in patient and doctor assessed symptom scores." Since this was a double-blind placebo-controlled study, you can't attribute the improvement to the placebo effect. As odd as it may be, homeopathy seems to work, at least for some conditions. A recent study published in the *British Medical Journal*, however, found that homeopathy worked no better than a placebo in the treatment of asthma.

If you want to try a homeopathic remedy for allergy, I recommend that you work with a homeopathic practitioner to get the best result. Naturopathic Doctors (NDs) are skilled in homeopathy, and are best equipped to steer you to the right treatment. Some complementary physicians may also have an expertise in homeopathy. Although it's difficult to self-treat with homeopathic remedies, there are some homeopathic combination antiallergy products on the market that take the guesswork out for consumers and are manufactured by well-known homeopathic companies such as Bioron and NatraBio. Orthodox homeopathic practitioners may not approve of this approach, preferring to custom-make each treatment for each patient, but these products do work for many people. If you want a more personalized approach, some natural food stores and pharmacies may have experts who understand homeopathy and can help you select the best product for you. For example, the Santa Monica Homeopathic Pharmacy in Santa Monica, California, offers counseling by qualified physicians who steer clients to the right remedies. There are also some excellent books on homeopathy for consumers.

HYPNOTHERAPY

Hypnotherapy is another form of alternative medicine that is becoming popular as a treatment for many different ailments, including asthma and allergy. The term hypnosis is from the Greek word "to sleep," but in reality, hypnosis has little to do with sleep and more to do with the power of the mind. Hypnosis is somewhat difficult to explain because it is still considered a mysterious phenomenon that is not fully understood. Nevertheless, there is a growing body of medical practitioners who recognize that it has value.

In hypnotherapy, a skilled practitioner guides you into a trancelike or meditative state in which you are trained to use your own thoughts to alter your physical state. The hypnotherapist is not controlling you or taking over your psyche, rather he or she is bringing you to the point where you are open to suggestions. Despite the popular image of the Svengalilike hypnotherapist manipulating his subject, in reality, under hypnosis, you won't do anything that you don't want to do. How does this work for allergy? When you are put in a hypnotic state, you are aware, but are also very relaxed and highly receptive to suggestions. If you believe that there is a body-mind connection, then it should be possible for your brain to "suggest" specific changes to different body systems. For example, several studies have documented that it is possible to boost immune function simply by thinking about rallying your immune cells to your defense. In fact, the practice of "guided imagery" is common among cancer patients and chronically ill patients. If our thoughts can boost a sluggish immune system, practitioners of hypnotherapy reason that our thoughts can normalize an overactive immune system, as in the case of allergy. This may sound a bit far-fetched, but in fact, a few studies have confirmed that people can dampen their allergic response to a substance when they are under hypnosis. In these studies, typically an allergen is injected into both arms, but the subject is told under hypnosis that only one arm will have an allergic reaction. In many of these experiments, the designated allergic arm showed a much greater allergic response than the other arm.

It is well-documented that guided visualization can actually cause an allergy attack. For example, if someone is highly allergic to cats, merely thinking about a cat is enough to trigger an allergic response. This is an example of letting the power of your mind work against you. On the other hand, hypnotherapy teaches you how to tap that power to work for you.

If you are interested in hypnotherapy for allergy or asthma, you should work with a well-trained hypnotherapist. To find the right person for you, contact the American Society of Clinical Hypnosis at 630-351-8489 or check out their website at www.asch.net. Hypnosis is not for everyone. Although most people are able to get to the point where they can let go and be open to suggestion, about 10 to 15 percent are not good candidates. Once you know how to get yourself into a hypnotic trance, you may be able to continue the therapy on your own.

YOGA

The practice of yoga, which originated more than five thousand years ago in India, is a spiritual practice that, in modern terms, combines the best of mind/body medicine. Yoga is derived from the Ayurvedic system of medicine that emphasizes treatment of the whole person, not simply the symptoms. In particular, Ayurvedic practitioners stress the importance of nutrition, a healthy body, and a tranquil mind. Practitioners of yoga called yogis aim to achieve true enlightenment, which they believe comes from the union with a divine consciousness known as Brahman or Atman, the transcendental self. In fact, the word yoga literally means "union" in Sanskrit, the ancient language of India. Ayurvedic medicine has provided a model for Western-style complementary medicine that combines conventional medicine with so-called alternative medicine—the use of therapies other than drugs.

There are many different forms of yoga, each with a different philosophical underpinning and approach. The practice of yoga typically consists of three components: (1) postures or asanas that promote strength, flexibility, and stamina; (2) breathing exercises called pranayama that strengthen lung function and promote relaxation; and (3) meditation, which helps to relieve stress, clear the mind, and achieve the loftier spiritual goals. Some forms of yoga may emphasize one aspect of yoga over the others. In recent years, yoga has become popular in the West as a way to stay calm and fit in a stressful world. Recent studies have shown that yoga is an excellent way to stay healthy and is actually being studied seriously by the medical community as an adjuvant treatment for many different problems ranging from arthritis to backache to high blood pressure to anxiety disorders. The National Institutes of Health (NIH) is funding clinical trials for yoga as a treatment for insomnia and multiple sclerosis.

Recent studies suggest that yoga is a useful therapy for asthma. In one study conducted at the University of Colorado, in Denver, an allergist studied seventeen adults with asthma. Half the group did a yoga regimen that included slow, deep breathing exercises and meditation, the other half did not. Those patients who did the yoga reported that they were less likely to use their inhalers than the control group, and they scored higher on quality-of-life questionnaires. Yoga did not improve lung function, but it did appear to improve symptoms and may lessen the need for strong medicine. In a different study conducted at the Institute for Respiratory Medicine in Australia, researchers investigated whether a particular meditation technique, Sahaja Yoga, could help asthmatics. The results were quite positive—asthma patients who did the yoga-style meditation showed a greater reduction in airway hyper-responsiveness (that is, overreaction to harmless substances) than did the control group. The results were published in *Thorax,* a leading peer review medical journal for respiratory health. Other studies have shown similar results.

Yoga advocates contend that yoga helps bring the body back to balance and that it can correct an overactive immune system, which should help allergy symptoms. If you are interested in trying yoga, you should find a class where you can work with a knowledgeable teacher who is aware of your particular health concerns. The website www.yoga.com is a great place to begin. It will give you basic information on yoga, as well as lists of teachers and classes in your area. Some forms of yoga, particularly the popular Power Yoga offered by many health clubs, can be hard on a weak back or a bad knee. If you have any orthopedic problems, check with your physician, chiropractor, or natural healer before beginning a yoga regimen. If you have asthma, be sure to work with someone who understands the problems of asthmatics. If done incorrectly, breathing exercises can do more harm than good.

CHAPTER 14

Traveling with Allergies

YOU'VE SPENT WEEKS PLANNING THE PERFECT VACATION. You've carefully researched the local entertainment, the cultural spots, and the best antique shops, and you can't wait to get away. Finally, you check into the quaint country inn that was recommended by your best friend, and it's everything he said it would be. Great location. Sensational views. Friendly owners. The problem is, there are a few things that he didn't tell you about. Like the owner is a cat lover, and his three cats are allowed to roam freely throughout the house—not so great for your cat allergy. Or that the inn allows smoking—not so great for your tobacco allergy. Or that the chef specializes in Thai cuisine—not so great for your peanut allergy. My point is, if you suffer from food or environmental allergies, your dream vacation can quickly turn into a nightmare.

Planning is your best defense against an all-out allergy attack on what should be a peaceful, enjoyable, *healthy* vacation. Here are some important tips on what you need to know to avoid ending up in allergy hell.

HAVE POLLEN SEASON WILL TRAVEL

As vegetation and climate varies throughout the world, so does pollen season. It may be freezing in New England, but parts of the southwestern United States may be starting to bloom. If you suffer from seasonal allergies, make sure that you're not unwittingly booking your vacation during the height of allergy season. If you want to know more about local pollen seasons and daily pollen counts, check out the following website: http://www.intellicast.com/Travel/.

If pollution bothers your allergies, don't forget to check out the air quality of your destination before booking your trip. Your lungs need a vacation too!

The beach is a great place to escape a pollen allergy—ocean breezes send pollen out to sea. Tired of the beach? Consider a cruise ship—but do get a smoke-free cabin.

BOOKING YOUR ROOM

Allergy proof your hotel room: If you've devoted time and expense to allergy proofing your bedroom, you shouldn't have to pay good money to stay in a room at a hotel or inn that is going to make you sick. When you make your reservation, tell the reservations clerk that you have allergies, and that you need to stay in a pet-free, smoke-free room. In addition, ask about the type of bedding used in the rooms—some people are allergic to feather pillows and down comforters, others may have problems with latex mattresses. If you are sensitive to strong chemical odors, you can ask that the cleaning staff use odor-free products.

Many hotels will be quite accommodating. In fact, one chain, Best Inn Suites and Hotels, offers environmentally friendly rooms featuring air purifiers, water filters, and special filter shower heads.

Survival tools: Bring a pillow protector to shield you from dust mites, and a mattress cover if you are staying for more than a few days and are very sensitive to dust mites. Bring your own disposable dust cloths to keep the room dust-free. If the hotel doesn't supply one, invest in a small room air purifier.

Special allergy alert: If you are allergic to peanuts, or have a severe food allergy to anything else, be sure that there are no offending foods or drinks lurking in the minibar.

PLANES, TRAINS, AND AUTOMOBILES

Emergency medicine: If you are at risk of a life-threatening allergic reaction and need to carry an epinephrine auto injector with you at all times, you will need to get security clearance to carry it on board, or it will be confiscated along with other sharp objects. Call the airlines ahead of time to see precisely what the airline requires of you in terms of documentation from your physician or a copy of your prescription, or you may not be able to bring your medication with you. If you have serious asthma and may require oxygen in the air, be sure to alert the airlines ahead of time. More important, before boarding, be sure that the airline attendants understand your medical needs and can assist you during an emergency.

Peanut alert: If you have a serious peanut allergy, check that the airline offers a peanut-free flight. Although "peanut-free" means that the flight attendants will not be handing out bags of mixed nuts with peanuts with beverage service, there is no guarantee that a passenger won't bring peanuts on board. Bring unscented wipes on board to clean off your food tray and the area surrounding your seat.

Bring your own food: I don't recommend eating anything prepared on an airplane, unless you are lucky enough to be sitting in first or business class where the menus are a bit more appetizing, and it's actually possible to get a reasonably healthy meal. If you have a food allergy, call ahead and see if you can order a special meal that does not contain your allergen. If you have serious food allergy, however, you need to be concerned about potential cross-contamination. Unlike a restaurant where you can speak directly to the chef, in this case, you really don't know for certain how a meal is prepared. Therefore, your best bet is to pack your own food.

Consider a portable air purifier: If you hate breathing stale airplane air, you can do something about it. You can wear a personal air purifier that hangs around your neck. It won't clean up the airplane cabin, but it can help clear out some pollutants and irritants in your immediate area. It's also useful for cars, trains, and subways. The only downside is that you may get some funny looks from the people sitting next to you.

Protect your ears: Under the best of circumstances, many people suffer from "airplane ear," a usually benign condition caused by changes in air pressure during takeoff and landing. The discomfort is caused by an air pocket inside the head that is vulnerable to changes in pressure. In many cases, chewing gum or frequent swallowing can help clear your ears—you may even feel them "pop" as the air pressure within the ear is normalized. However, airplane ear can be aggravated by an existing cold, allergy, or sinus infection. The sinus membranes are connected to the inner ear by the eustachian tube, a small, thin, narrow structure. When the sinus membranes get swollen—as they do during a cold or an allergy attack—they can block the middle ear, causing fluid in the ear. The combination of an already irritated middle ear and airplane travel can not be only be painful, but can be dangerous and can lead to injury of the eardrum. If you are very congested, it's best not to fly, if possible. However, if you must fly, talk to your doctor about using an antihistamine or decongestant before takeoff and possibly before landing (depending on the length of the flight) to help clear out your sinuses and reduce swelling. People who have high blood pressure, heart disease, or thyroid conditions should not use many of the over-the-counter antihistamines. Ask your physician about products that may be safe for you. And please don't get in the habit of using antihistamines—they can have undesirable side effects, and they lose their effectiveness fairly quickly if you overuse them.

Smoke-free transportation: Although all flights originating in the United States are now smoke-free, overseas it's a different story. If you're booking a foreign airline, be sure to specify that you want to be on a smoke-free flight. If you're taking the train, make sure that it has a smoke-free section. Most commuter and long-distance trains in the United States are smoke-free, although some may have a smokers' car. In Europe, where smoking is rampant, you may have to specifically book a seat in a nonsmoking section. And if you rent a car on your trip, don't forget to tell the reservation clerk that you want a smoke-free car.

Eating out: When you are away from home, particularly in a foreign country, you have to be very careful about food allergy. It's easy for a mishap to occur if you're not fluent in the language. If you have a potentially life-threatening food allergy, be sure to have someone who speaks the language write down your food requirements on a small card you can put in your wallet and show to the waiter or the chef. If you are unfamiliar with an ingredient in a particular dish, or it's doused in a mystery sauce, don't eat it. Ordering simple food, as close as possible to its natural state, is safer (and actually, a lot healthier!). When you travel, it's very important to wear a medic alert bracelet so that people know you have a serious allergy that may require medical attention.

YOUR MEDICINE

I am hoping that by following my advice, many of you will require less medication, and possibly no medication. However, if you still use medication for allergy or asthma, be sure to pack enough for the entire trip. Keep your medicine in its original bottles or you may run into trouble at Customs. In addition, it's a good idea to carry an extra copy of your prescriptions with you should you need more medicine, or encounter a suspicious Customs officer. Have your doctor give you the name of a physician you can contact if you have a problem.

Resources

The following companies or organizations will provide information on products and services mentioned in this book.

Allergy Control Products, Inc.
Wide variety of products to allergy proof your home.
96 Danbury Road
Ridgefield, CT 06877
1-800-422-DUST (3878)
www.allergycontrol.com

Allergyreliefstore.com
Wide variety of products to allergy proof your home.

EDDIE BAUER
eddiebauer.com
1-800-625-7935
Offers nonallergenic alternatives to down blankets and pillows.

www.foodallergy.org
Provides comprehensive information on food allergy and
related products. This is an excellent source of
information, especially for parents of allergic kids.

GAIAM HARMONY
Natural cotton clothing, nontoxic cleansing products.
www.gaiam.com
1-800-869-3446

www.greenmarketplace.com
Supplier of environmentally friendly, nontoxic products
for the home.
1-888-59-EARTH

HAMMACHER SCHLEMMER
www.hammacher.com
147 E. 57th Street
New York, NY
1-800-421-9002
Sells air purifiers for home and office.

LAND'S END
landsend.com
1-800-356-4444
Offers nonallergenic alternatives to down blankets and
pillows.

www.shop.store.yahoo.com/hemp-organic/
Where to buy natural cotton and organic clothes.

SEVENTH GENERATION

Great source of nontoxic, environmentally friendly products. Offers their own brand of cleansers and paper products sold by catalogue, on the Internet, or in stores.
1-800-456-1191
www.seventhgeneration.com

SHARPER IMAGE

Great source for home and office air purifiers.
www.sharperimage.com
1-800-344-4444

Bibliography

"Allergies to Animals." *Medfacts*. National Jewish Medical and Research Center, Denver.

"Asthma and Allergy Statistics." National Institute of Allergy and Infectious Disease. Office of Communications and Public Liaison, Bethesda, Md.

"Asthma Triggers." U.S. Environmental Protection Agency, Washington, D.C., 2002.

Bardana, E., and Montanaro, A., eds. *Annals of Allergy, Asthma & Immunology:* 83: (6) Suppl-Occupational Asthma and Allergies (entire issue: December 1999).

Barilla, J., et al. *The Nutrition Superbook: The Antioxidants,* Vol 1. Keats Publishing, New Canaan, Conn., 1995.

Bauer, K., et al. "Pharmacodynamic Effects of Inhaled Dry Powder Formulations of Feneterol and Colforsin in Asthma." *Clin Pharmacol Ther.* 43:76–83, 1993.

Beers, M. H., and Fletcher, A. J. *The Merck Manual,* 17th edition. Merck & Co., Inc., Whitehouse Station, N.J., 1999.

Bendich, A., and Langseth, L. "The Health Effects of Vitamin C Supplementation: A Review." *Journal of the American College of Nutrition:* 14:124–36.

Billups, N. F., ed. *American Drug Index 2002*, 45th edition. Billups Facts and Comparisons, St. Louis, Mo., 2002.

Chari, P., et al. "Acupuncture Therapy in Allergic Rhinitis." *American Journal of Acupuncture:* 16 (2):43–147 (April–June 1988).

Clark, D. G., and Wyatt, Kate. *Colostrum: Life's First Food.* CNR Publications, Salt Lake City, 1996.

Collipp, P. J., et al. "Pyridozine Treatment of Childhood Bronchial Asthma." *Ann Allergy:* 35:93–97 (1975).

De Flora, S., Grassi, C., and Carati, L. "Attenuation of Flu-Like Symptomatology and Improvement in Cell Mediated Immunity with Long Term N-acetylcysteine Treatment." *European Respiratory Journal:* 10:1535–41 (1997).

Dorsch, W., et al. "Antiasthmatic Effects of Onions. Inhibition of Platelet-Activating Factor-Induced Bronchial Obstruction by Onion Oils." *International Archives of Allergy and Applied Immunology:* 82 (3–4):535–36 (1987).

Durlach, J. "Magnesium Depletion, Magnesium Deficiency and Asthma." *Magnesium Research:* 8:403–5 (1995).

Fenrich, J., and Vidaurri, V. "Psoriasis." *International Journal of Pharmaceutical Compounding:* 4 (5):348–56 (September–October 2000).

Fleming, T. *Physicians' Desk Reference for Herbal Medicines,* 2nd edition 2000. Medical Economics, Montvale, N.J., 2002.

"Food Allergy." *U.S. Pharmacist:* February 2002, HS41–43.

"Food Allergy and Intolerance." National Institute of Allergy and Infectious Disease. Office of Communications and Public Liaisons. National Institutes of Health, Washington, D.C., June 2001.

Fulder, S., and Blackwood, J. *Garlic: Nature's Original Remedy.* Healing Arts Press, Rochester, Vt., 1991.

Gaby, A. *Magnesium: How an Important Mineral Helps Prevent Heart Attacks and Relieve Stress.* Keats Publishing, New Canaan, Conn., 1994.

Gergen, G., et al. "The Prevalence of Allergic Skin Reactivity to Eight Common Allergens in the U.S. Population: Results from the Second National Health and Nutrition Examination Survey." *J Allergy Clinical Immunol:* 800:669–79 (1987).

Gupta, I., et al. "Effects of Boswellia Serrata Gum Resin in Patients with Bronchial Asthma: Results of a Double Blind Placebo Controlled, 6-Week Clinical Study." *Eur J Med Res:* 3:511–14 (1998).

Gupta, S., et al. "Tylophora Indica in Bronchial Asthma—a Doubleblind Study." *Ind Journ Med Res:* 69:981–89 (1979).

Hamilton, G. "Let Them Eat Dirt." *New Scientist:* July 18, 1998.

Hardman, J., and Limbird, L. E. *Goodman and Gillman's The Pharmacological Basis of Therapeutics,* 10th edition. McGraw-Hill Health Professions Division, New York, 2001.

Hasselmark, L., et al. "Selenium Supplementation in Intrinsic Asthma." *Allergy:* 48:30–36 (1993).

Hederos, C. A., and Berg. A. "Epogram Evening Primrose

Oil Treatment in Atopic Dermatitis and Asthma." *Archives of Disease in Childhood:* 75:494–97 (1996).

Hepintal, S., et al. "Extracts of Feverfew Inhibit Granule Secretion in Blood Platelets and Polymorphonuclear Leucocytes." *The Lancet:* 1071–73 (May 11, 1985).

Hobbs, C. "Sarsaparilla, A Literature Review." *Herbal-Gram:* No. 17 (1988).

Houseini, S., et al. "Pycnogenol in the Management of Asthma." *Journal of Medicinal Food:* 4 (4):201–8 (2001).

"Indoor Air Facts No. 8: Use and Care of Home Humidifiers." U.S. Environmental Protection Agency, Washington, D.C., 1991.

"Indoor Air Quality." U.S. Environmental Protection Agency, Washington, D.C., 2002.

Jaret, P. "The Antibiotic Crisis." *Hippocrates:* 12:26–33 (1998).

Kellman, R. *Gut Reactions.* Broadway Books, New York, 2002.

Kelly, G. "Clinical Applications of N-acetylcysteine." *Alternative Medicine Review:* 114–27 (1998).

Kessinger, J. "Allergies: The Controversy." *The Original Internist:* 2–3 (September 2001).

Kleijenen, J., et al. "Acupuncture and Asthma: A Review of Controlled Trials." *Thorax:* 46:799–802 (1991).

Koltai, M., et al. "Platelet Activating Factor (PAF): A Review of its Effects, Antagonists and Possible Future Clinical Implications" (Part I). *Drugs:* 42 (1):9–29 (1991).

Leung, A. Y., and Foster, S. *Encyclopedia of Common Natural Ingredients Used in Food.* John Wiley & Sons, New York, 1996.

Majeed, M., et al. *Turmeric and the Healing Curcuminoids.* Keats Publishing, New Canaan, Conn., 1996.

Manacha, R., et al. "Sahaja Yoga in the Management of Moderate to Severe Asthma: A Randomised Controlled Trial." *Thorax:* 57:110–15 (2002).

Middleton, E., and Drzewiecki, G. "Quercetin: An Inhibitor of Antigen-Induced Human Basophil Histamine Release." *Int. Archs Allergy Appl Immunology:* 77:155–57 (1985).

Mindell, Earl. *Earl Mindell's New Herb Bible.* Fireside, New York, 2000.

————. *The Power of MSM.* Contemporary Books, New York, 2002.

Mittman, R. "Randomized, Double-Blind Study of Freezedried Urtica Dioica in the Treatment of Allergic Rhinitis." *Planta Medica:* 56:44–47 (1990).

Mowrey, D. *The Scientific Validation of Herbal Medicine.* Keats Publishing, New Canaan, Conn., 1986.

Nagakura, T., et al. "Dietary Supplementation with Fish Oil Rich in Omega-3 Polyunsaturated Fatty Acids in Children with Bronchial Asthma." *Eur Respir J:* 16:861–65 (2000).

Naturopathic Handbook of Herbal Formulas. Herbal Research Publications Inc., Ayer, Mass., 1995.

Okamoto, M., et al. "Effects of Dietary Supplementation with n-3 Fatty Acids Compared with n-6 Fatty Acids on Bronchial Asthma." *Intern Med:* 39 (2):107–11 (February 2000).

O'Neil, M. J. *The Merck Index,* 13th edition. Merck & Co., Inc. Whitehouse Station, N.J., 2001.

Packer, L., and Colman, C. *The Antioxidant Miracle: Your*

Complete Plan for Total Health and Healing. John Wiley & Sons, New York, 1999.

Packer, L., et al. *Vitamin C in Health and Disease.* Marcel Dekker, New York, 1997.

Park, Alice. "A Kiss Before Sneezing." *Time:* June 17, 2002.

Passwater, R. A. *All About Selenium.* Avery Publishing Group, New York, 1999.

Pauling, L. *How to Live Longer and Feel Better.* Avon Books, New York, 1987.

Pelton, R., et al. *Drug-Induced Nutrient Depletion Handbook.* Lexi Comp, Inc., Hudson, Ohio, 2001.

Reilly, D. T., et al. "Is Homeopathy a Placebo Response?" *The Lancet:* 881–86 (October 18, 1986).

Rice-Evans, C., and Packer, L. *Flavonoids in Health and Disease.* Marcel Dekker, New York, 1997.

Romeiu, I. "Antioxidant Supplementation and Respiratory Functions Among Workers Exposed to High Levels of Ozone." *Am J Respir Crit Care Med:* 158:226–32 (1998).

Rountree, R., et al. *Immunotics: Your Personal Immune Boosting Program.* P. P. Putnam & Sons, New York, 2000.

Rylander, R., et al. "Magnesium Supplementation Decreases Airway Responsiveness Among Hyperactive Subjects." *Magnesium-Bulletin:* 19:4–6 (1997).

Schapowal, A. "Randomized Controlled Trial of Butterbur and Cetirizine for Treating Seasonal Allergic Rhinitis." *British Medical Journal:* 324:144 (January 19, 2002).

Shahani, K., and Ayebo, A. "Role of Dietary Lactobacilli in Gastrointestinal Microecology." *American Journal of Clinical Nutrition:* 33:2448–57 (1980).

Shaheen, S. O., et al. "Dietary Antioxidants and Asthma in Adults." *Am J Crit Care Med:* 164:1823–28 (2001).

Shirota, M. "What You Should Know About Medicinal Mushrooms." *Explore!:* 48–49 (1996).

Shute, Nancy. "Allergy Epidemic." *U.S. News & World Report,* May 5, 2000.

Sifton, D. W., *Physicians' Desk Reference 2002,* 56th edition. Medical Economics, Inc., Montvale, N.J., 2002.

———. *Physicians' Desk Reference for OTC Drugs 2002.* Medical Economics, Montvale, N.J., 2002.

Simopoulos, A. "Omega-3 Fatty Acids in Health and Disease and in Growth and Development." *American Journal of Clinical Nutrition:* 54:438–63 (1991).

Sinatra, S. *The Coenzyme Q10 Phenomenon.* Keats Publishing, New Canaan, Conn., 1998.

"State of the Air 2002 Report." American Lung Association, Washington, D.C., 2002.

Sussman, G. L., and Breezehold, D. H. "Allergy to Latex Rubber." *Annals of Internal Medicine:* 122:43–46 (1995).

Taussig, S. J., and Batkin, S. "Bromelain, the Enzyme Complex of Pineapple (Ananas cosmosus) and Its Clinical Application." *Journal of Ethnopharmacology:* 22:191–203 (1988).

Teguaruden, R. *Chinese Tonic Herbs.* Japan Publications, Inc., Tokyo and New York, 1987.

Tierney, L. M., McPhee, S. J., and Papadakis, M. Lange. *Current Medical Diagnosis and Treatment 2002,* 41st edition. McGraw-Hill, New York, 2002.

Ullman, R., and Reichenberg-Ullman, J. *Homeopathic Self-Care.* Prima Publishing, Rocklin Ca., 1997.

Wagner, H. "Search for New Plant Constituents with Potential Antiphlogistic and Antiallergic Activity." *Planta Medica:* 55:235–41 (1989).

Welton, A. F., et al. "Effect of Flavonoids on Arachnidonic Acid Metabolism." *Prog Clin Biol Res:* 213:231–42 (1986).

"What is Eczema?" American Academy of Dermatology. Schaumburg, Illinois.

Winter, Greg. "Calls Increasing for Clarity on Food Labels." *New York Times,* July 2, 2002.

Zand, J., Walton, R., and Rountree, B. *Smart Medicine for a Healthier Child.* Avery Press, Garden City, N.Y., 1994.

Ziment, I., and Tashkin, D. "Alternative Medicine for Allergy and Asthma." *J Allergy Clin Immuno:* 106:603–14 (October 2000).

Zimmerman, Marcia. "Immune Enhancers." *Nutrition Science News:* 4:84–90 (1999).

———. "Zinc Lozenges Reduce Duration of Common Cold Symptoms." *Nutr Rev:* 55:82–88 (1997).

Index

Main entries for supplements, medications, treatments, and specific allergies appear in bold type.